THE
EVIDENCE-BASED
PRACTICE MANUAL
FOR NURSES

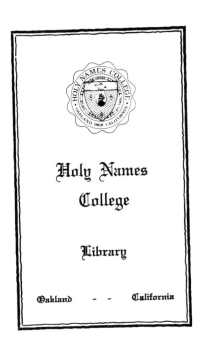

Holy Names
College

Library

Oakland - - California

For *Churchill Livingstone*

Commissioning Editor: Sarena Wolfaard
Project Development Manager: Karen Gilmour
Project Manager: Jane Dingwall
Design Direction: Judith Wright

THE EVIDENCE-BASED PRACTICE MANUAL FOR NURSES

Edited by

Jean V Craig MSc RSCN RGN

Research Associate, Evidence-Based Child Health Unit, University of Liverpool, Institute of Child Health, Alder Hey Children's Hospital, Liverpool, UK

Rosalind L Smyth MA MBBS MD MRCP DCH FRCPCH

Brough Professor of Paediatric Medicine, University of Liverpool, Institute of Child Health, Alder Hey Children's Hospital, Liverpool, UK

Foreword by
Sarah Mullally
Chief Nursing Officer, Department of Health, London, UK

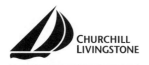

Edinburgh London New York Oxford Philadelphia St Louis Sydney Toronto 2002

CHURCHILL LIVINGSTONE
An imprint of Elsevier Science Limited

First published 2002
  Reprinted 2002, 2003

ISBN 0 443 07064 4

British Library Cataloguing in Publication Data
A catalogue record for this book is available from the British Library.

Library of Congress Cataloging in Publication Data
A catalog record for this book is available from the Library of Congress.

Note
Medical knowledge is constantly changing. As new information becomes
available, changes in treatment, procedures, equipment and the use of drugs
become necessary. The editors, contributors and the publishers have taken
care to ensure that the information given in this text is accurate and up to date.
However, readers are strongly advised to confirm that the information,
especially with regard to drug usage, complies with the latest legislation and
standards of practice.

 your source for books,
journals and multimedia
in the health sciences
www.elsevierhealth.com

Printed in China
B/03

Contents

Contributors

Editors

Jean V Craig (Chapters 1 and 2) Research Associate, Evidence-Based Child Health Unit, University of Liverpool, Institute of Child Health, Alder Hey Children's Hospital, Liverpool, UK

Rosalind L Smyth (Chapter 7) Brough Professor of Paediatric Medicine, Institute of Child Health, University of Liverpool, Alder Hey Children's Hospital, Liverpool, UK

Contributors

Olwen Beaven (Chapter 3) Information Specialist, Clinical Evidence, BMJ Publishing Group, BMA House, London, UK

Rhona Hotchkiss (Chapters 8 and 11) Nursing and Midwifery Practice Development Unit, Elliot House, Edinburgh, UK

Ann Jacoby (Chapter 6) Professor of Medical Sociology, Department of Primary Care, University of Liverpool, Liverpool, UK

Mark Learmonth (Chapter 9) Lecturer in Health and Social Care Management, The University of York, York, UK

Andrea Litva (Chapter 6) Lecturer in Medical Sociology, Department of Primary Care, University of Liverpool, Liverpool, UK

Mark Newman (Chapters 4 and 5) ESRC Research Fellow/Senior Lecturer, School of Health, Biological and Environmental Sciences, School of Life Long Learning and Education, Middlesex University, London, UK

Maggie Pearson (Chapter 1) Professor of Health and Community Care, University of York, York, UK

Lin Perry (Chapter 10) Senior Researcher, Faculty of Health and Social Care Sciences, Grosvenor Wing, St George's Hospital Medical School, London, UK

Tony Roberts (Chapters 4 and 5) Research Fellow in Public Health, South Tees Hospital NHS Trust, North Tees Primary Care Trust and The University of Durham, Middlesbrough, UK

Mandie Sunderland (Chapter 11) Director of Nursing and Quality, Blackpool Victoria Hospital, NHS Trust, Blackpool, UK

Lois Thomas (Chapter 8) Senior Lecturer in Research, University of Central Lancashire, Preston, UK

Carl Thompson (Chapter 9) Centre for Evidence-Based Nursing, University of York, York, UK

Foreword

Nurses are committed to delivering high-quality care that meets the needs of their patients, but it is in identifying and indeed recognising what constitutes high quality that the challenge lies.

Nurses are rising to this challenge. They are increasingly listening to, and working with, their patients to identify what it is they want from the health service. They accept that it is no longer acceptable to purely base practice on tradition. Practice must be continuously reviewed, continuously questioned and, where appropriate, decisions made based upon available evidence.

This evidence is not purely focused upon clinical interventions and therapies but, as nursing research continues to flourish, relates to all aspects of health, health care and the patient experience. Therefore, many types of evidence from many sources will need to be considered. This will require nurses to develop or utilise an array of skills, to not only review the evidence but to then apply it to their practice. This is where this manual provides that practical support.

Through the use of real life examples it will help individual nurses in their efforts to achieve an evidence-based approach to clinical practice, supporting them in asking the right questions, developing the skills they need to explore and evaluate evidence, all to the eventual benefit of the patients. Developed by leading researchers and clinicians the manual provides a very valuable tool for your personal professional development. I commend it to you.

Sarah Mullally

Preface

'Evidence-based' is one of the most used, and perhaps least understood, adjectives in health care today. It was previously applied almost exclusively in the term 'evidence-based medicine', but happily terms such as 'evidence-based practice' are becoming more widespread and emphasise that this is a concept that should apply to all of health care. Nurses, the largest group of professionals who provide health care, have been at the forefront in recognising the need to identify, evaluate and apply best evidence to their clinical practice. However, not all may feel that they have the skills and knowledge to do this. We believe that with the help of this manual, nurses will be able to apply the techniques of evidence-based practice in their own individual settings.

The manual is divided into three sections: section 1 provides the background and context for the evidence-based 'movement' in nursing and gives details of some of the challenges (and solutions) that nursing as a profession, and individual nurses, are faced with when trying to ensure that patient care is informed by scientific evidence.

Section 2 focuses on the practical skills required for identifying best evidence to support health care decisions. It provides detailed, step-by-step guidance in formulating focused clinical questions (an important skill, as it is the question that drives each subsequent step of the process), in conducting successful searches of electronic databases, and in critically appraising research studies that use qualitative or quantitative methods. It also provides a grounding in the conduct and interpretation of systematic reviews and meta-analyses, and highlights the importance of this form of research in informing best patient care.

Section 3 focuses on how to make evidence-based practice a reality. The role of guidelines as a method for implementing best evidence is considered, and the reader is provided with tools for assessing their rigour. A step-by-step approach is used to guide the reader through the process of implementing change in practice.

The practical strategies that organisations need to consider if they are to promote and sustain an evaluative, evidence-based approach to their work are discussed, and health care policies are explored in the light of research evidence.

We have provided a glossary of useful terms at the end of the manual and, for nurses wishing to further develop their knowledge and skills, a list of books and other resources that we have found to be useful can be found in the Further Reading sections at the end of each chapter.

Finally, we emphasise that the skills taught in this book must be integrated with clinical skills and expertise to ensure high-quality nursing care. Nurses, as a profession, are uniquely placed to understand patients' needs, priorities and beliefs and to integrate these considerations with their own expertise and with clinical evidence in making decisions.

Jean V Craig
Rosalind L Smyth

Section 1

THE CONTEXT FOR EVIDENCE-BASED PRACTICE

1

Evidence-based practice in nursing

Maggie Pearson and Jean V Craig

Key points

- An evidence-based approach to clinical practice aims to deliver appropriate care in an efficient manner to individual patients.
- The process entails the integration of research evidence, clinical expertise and the interpretation of patients' needs and perspectives in making decisions.
- Nursing care involves a wide range of interventions and therefore draws on a diverse evidence base (including, for example, evidence from psychology, sociology and public health).
- Individual nurses need to develop key skills in order to access and use evidence appropriately in clinical practice and, where evidence is not available, to make considered decisions.
- Sources of synthesised evidence are evolving and are being made accessible to nurses.
- In terms of developing nurse researchers, issues such as organisational culture, management support, and career paths that accommodate both clinical and research work need to be addressed.

Introduction

At the heart of the UK government's drive to modernise health care is a commitment to the development of quality, person-centred health services based on evidence (Department of Health 1997). The strategy for nursing, *Making a Difference* (Department of Health 1999), reflects this commitment, and emphasises the need for a robust evidence base for nursing, midwifery and health visiting. The vision for nursing in the twenty-first century is for all nurses to seek out evidence and apply it in their everyday practice, with an increasing proportion actively participating in research and development, and some developing into research leaders (Department of Health 2000a).

Evidence-based health care: what is it and why do we need it?

Within the campaign to improve the quality of health care, there is a great deal of talk about 'evidence-based practice'. This phrase trips lightly off the tongue, and can engender a reassuring warm glow that all is well: we know what needs to be done, and all that is required is for practitioners to implement the evidence. If only it were that simple!

Evidence-based practice has been described as 'doing the right things right' (Muir Gray 1997, page 18). This means not only doing things more efficiently and to the best standard possible, but also ensuring that that which *is* done, is done 'right' – so that more good than harm results.

Intuitively, few practitioners would disagree with this approach, but there are several hurdles on the way to this goal: we need the evidence base to know what it is 'right' to do; we have to be clear to whom the evidence really applies; and we also have to be clear at what stage in a person's trajectory of health or illness the evidence-based intervention is indicated. All this, at a time when the pressures are increasing to deliver challenging service targets, to reduce waiting at all stages of the patient experience and to place the person at the centre of their health care (Department of Health 2000b). The key point here is that, if we can get it right, evidence-based practice *will* help to improve people's experiences of illness and health care, and good established nursing practice already does.

It is important to remember that whilst the phrase 'evidence-based practice' is relatively new in the everyday vocabulary of health interventions and health care, the concept itself is not new. We would be doing our predecessors a great disservice to pretend otherwise. Let us take two basic examples: infection control and prevention of deep vein thrombosis are key, long-established aspects of nursing care, undertaken daily in hospitals and in people's homes, which can prevent complications arising from immobility or vulnerability to infection. These long-established practices avoid 'unnecessary' distress, treatments, days immobilised at home or in hospital. Indeed, it is salutary to reflect that within England the number of hospital inpatient days attributed to hospital-acquired infection (HAI) has risen dramatically over the last 10 years (Department of Health 2001a). The associated economic burden is estimated to amount to at least £1 billion pounds a year (Plowman et al 1999, 2001). This increase in HAI is especially worrying, in view of the risk of antibiotic-resistant infections such as methicillin-resistant *Staphylococcus aureus*. Why this problem should be on the increase is not entirely clear, but factors such as falling hygiene standards within hospitals (Department of Health 2001a), and poor compliance with handwashing (Handwashing Liaison Group 1999) are possible contributors.

There is a particularly cruel irony in the rise of hospital-acquired infections in an era in which evidence-based practice is generally accepted as a key component of modern health care: perhaps one of the earliest documented examples of evidence-based practice was the development of aseptic technique in the nineteenth century, following observations of cross-infection. For example, in the 1840s, Semmelweis's insistence that doctors performing autopsies should wash their hands before going on to deliver babies was associated with a dramatic reduction in mortality due to sepsis from over a fifth to 3% (Rotter 1997). Similarly, it was careful observation that led John Snow (Figure 1.1) in the 1840s to pinpoint the cause of the outbreak of cholera in London to a water tap in Broad Street. These two examples from the nineteenth century encapsulate the breadth of domains of professional practice in health which can and should be evidence-based; but they also demonstrate powerfully how reflective, questioning and acutely observant practitioners can uncover evidence within their own everyday practice which, when acted upon, can improve health, although not all examples will be quite so dramatic!

John Snow's observation in respect of cholera serves to remind us that whilst the recent concept of 'evidence-based practice' first arose in hospital care for individual patients, it is as relevant and important in public health interventions and community development as in intensive care units. Indeed, the UK Economic and Social Research Council has recently invested in a network of research centres that will pull together the evidence base for public policy and its implementation. One of these, to be based at the MRC

Figure 1.1 **John Snow, English anaesthetist and epidemiologist. Photograph of oil painting by Thomas Jones Barker (1847). From the Wellcome Library, London, with permission. Videodisc no. 51428**

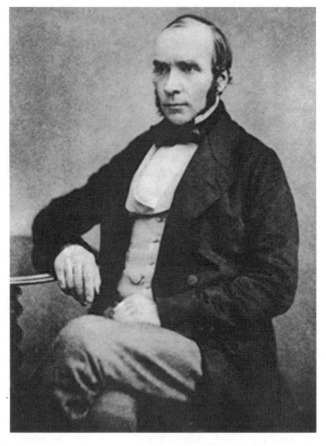

Medical Sociology Unit in Glasgow, will address the evidence base for non-health care interventions which improve health.

It is clear that no aspects of nursing practice for health, whether in the community, home or hospital, should be 'safe' from the concept of evidence-based practice. In some areas, acceptance of the concept is not the problem: but the reality is! In those (largely hospital clinical) areas where there has been a great deal of research, it is almost impossible to keep on top of the burgeoning body of knowledge that emerges daily, and the challenge is to be able to manage that knowledge so that busy practitioners can find it accessible and be alert to its quality. Amidst the mass of publications it is important to be able to discern how robust the evidence is: how the study was designed, and the extent to which the results can be generalised to a wider population. It is important to remember that different kinds of 'evidence' and knowledge are generated by different kinds of research methodologies: all have their place, but we need to be mindful of the strengths and weaknesses of each.

Furthermore, where we do have robust evidence, we need to be clear and careful about to whom it applies. It is crucial that evidence from clinical trials undertaken with a specific population subsample is not inappropriately extrapolated to other population subgroups. For example, the majority of clinical trials are undertaken in samples of people under the age of 65. Care should therefore be taken in extrapolating that evidence, which will of necessity have been generated in people with few co-morbidities that could 'confuse' the results, to older people who could have several co-existing conditions. Randomised controlled trials have shown, for example, that thrombolytic therapy significantly reduces the risk of death in patients with acute myocardial infarction (MI) (Fibrinolytic Therapy Trialists 1994), but only 10% of the sample populations in the trials were >74 years of age, and when the results for these participants were examined, the efficacy of the therapy was found to be ambiguous.

In other spheres of health-related interventions and health care, however, we simply do not have enough robust evidence to really know what it is 'right' to do. The priority is to generate the evidence required, but that takes time if it is to be done properly. So what should be done in the mean time? Where there is no robust evidence base, the ethos of evidence-based practice should, at the very least, stop us in our tracks to reflect on the impact of what we are doing in the name of health, and why. Reflective practice is a key component of evidence-based health care; the very ethos of good professional practice is to reflect on the taken-for-granted assumptions that underpin everyday practice, and to routinely assess the impact and outcomes of interactions and interventions with patients, clients and the public. And we need to do all this without becoming 'frozen' and disempowered by the lack of robust evidence for much of what we do.

The evidence-based movement across health care

In the early years of the evidence-based 'movement', the discourse was limited to 'medicine', rather than health care (Sackett et al 1997), but more recently the principles of evidence-based medicine have been applied to other spheres of professional practice in health and social care such as pharmacy (Tully & Cantrill 1999), complementary medicine (Lewith 1996), the therapies (Bury & Mead 1998), and orthodontics (Harrison 2000). Whereas the Cochrane Collaboration reviews and synthesises evidence on the impact of health care interventions, the Campbell Collaboration reviews and synthesises evidence of the impact of educational and social interventions.

Development of the evidence-based concept

The first textbook on evidence-based medicine (EBM) defined it as: 'the conscientious, explicit and judicious use of current best evidence in making decisions about the health care of patients' (Sackett et al 1997, page 2). The authors elaborated that the practice of EBM entailed the integration of individual clinical expertise with the best available external clinical evidence from systematic research, and involved taking account of the patient's perspective in making clinical decisions.

Contrary to the assertions of its critics, therefore, that EBM was narrowly concerned with the conduct of randomised controlled trials and the implementation of their results in routine practice (Grahame Smith 1998), the 'product champions' of EBM never argued that it was 'simply' a matter of slavishly following rigid guidelines based solely on the findings of clinical trials: the need to tailor care on the basis of research evidence and clinical experience to the needs of patients was always acknowledged.

In 2000, Sackett and colleagues included the value of clinical expertise and patient perspectives more explicitly in their definition of EBM as 'the integration of best research evidence with clinical expertise and patient values' (Sackett et al 2000, page 1).

They define their terms carefully:

■ *Best research evidence* is defined as

clinically relevant research, often from the basic sciences of medicine (sic), but especially from patient-centred clinical research. (Sackett et al 2000, page 1).

They go on to assert that

> New evidence from clinical research both invalidates previously accepted diagnostic tests and treatments and replaces them with new ones that are more powerful, more accurate, more efficacious and safer. (Sackett et al 2000, page 1)

Note that the discourse is about 'diagnostic tests' and 'treatments', whereas the broader concept of 'care' which embodies nursing practice in all settings involves much more: communication, comfort, observation for example. This means that, in applying these principles to the variety of nursing practice, we need to draw on a range of evidence bases in psychology, sociology, and possibly, for improving comfort, ergonomics!

■ *Clinical expertise* is defined as

> the ability to use our clinical skills and past experience to rapidly identify each patient's unique health state and diagnosis, their individual risks and benefits of potential interventions, and their personal values and expectations. (Sackett et al 2000, page 1).

Personal professional experience, clinical judgement and even intuition have a role to play.

■ By *'patient values'*, the authors mean:

> the unique preferences, concerns and expectations each patient brings to a clinical encounter and which must be integrated into clinical decisions if they are to serve the patient. (Sackett et al 2000, page 1).

In reality then, EBM is manifest not 'simply' by the implementation of 'patient centred clinical research', but by the integration of systematically derived research-based knowledge with the practitioner's tacit knowledge drawn from experience and their interpretation of the needs and perspectives of each person with whom they interact in individual clinical encounters. What is implied is that truly evidence-based practice must involve the patient in the clinical decisions.

The principles enunciated by Sackett and colleagues are clearly of direct relevance to all professional practice, but for any practitioner this is a daunting agenda. It means having access to an up-to-date synthesis of research findings in a form that can be assimilated, having confidence in one's own professional judgement and having the communication skills, insight and empathy to 'read' and respond to the patient's circumstances and needs. Narrowing the concept down to 'investigations and treatments' perhaps makes the concept and requisite evidence base more manageable, but the majority of nursing practice cannot retreat into such a focused definition. Nursing care involves a wider range of interventions and needs to draw on a wide range of research-based evidence. For example, whilst there is an emerging body of research-based evidence about how best to manage leg ulcers (Cullum et al 2001), nurses do not 'simply' treat leg ulcers: they care for the person with the leg ulcer.

Challenges

The challenge, then, for nursing practice (as for all professional practice) is to develop and draw on the well-focused evidence base relating to specific clinical treatments to improve the quality of clinical procedures, whilst also drawing on a more diverse evidence base for the wider concept of care which they provide (Pursey et al 1997). This challenge is not straightforward: if it is to become a reality rather than a vain but noble hope, there are several imperatives to be addressed. These will take both time and resources.

First, the relevant research-based evidence bases are not comprehensive: there are yawning gaps in the robust evidence for much of what nurses do in the course of their daily work. Rigorous research to address these gaps takes time, and established research expertise in nursing is in relatively short supply (Department of Health 1998b, Pearson 2000). It is important that the recognition of the needs for evidence-based practice does not result in a misguided and undiscerning dash to seek out *any* 'knowledge' available, irrespective of the quality of research on which it is based. Critical appraisal skills will be crucial to enable practitioners thirsty for knowledge to discriminate between high- and poor-quality evidence.

Secondly, the relevant evidence bases are not static: there has been an explosion in the volume of research publications over the last few decades and it is impossible for any busy practitioner to keep abreast of the literature. More than 74 000 health service research publications were produced in the UK alone in 1997 with an average annual growth rate of almost 4% (Wellcome Trust

2001). We urgently need effective means of synthesising the emerging evidence and making this updated knowledge base accessible. In England, the National Electronic Library for Health is intended to fulfil that function.

Thirdly, life-long learning is generally accepted as an important principle in the twenty-first century, not just for busy professionals who need to keep abreast of the knowledge in their field and adapt to role changes (Department of Health, 2001b), but for citizens generally, whose roles and opportunities in work and socially are constantly changing as the technological and social revolutions leave no holes barred. For professions such as those involved in health care, steeped in tradition and an ethos of established expertise, the notion that established procedures may not be based on robust evidence, or that new knowledge may challenge some established shibboleths is not comfortable. Furthermore, if busy practitioners are to have the time to access the evidence base and update their knowledge, there are clear human and financial resource implications: all at a time when recruitment and retention of staff are acknowledged to be key constraints which the service faces in meeting public expectations and increasingly challenging targets set by government.

Finally, the fact that a piece of research has been conducted does not automatically mean that the findings should be transferred directly into the clinical setting. Individual research studies need to be examined in the context of other evidence before a practice change is initiated. Consider, for example, the management of gastro-oesophageal reflux, a condition in which recurrent vomiting, failure to thrive, feeding difficulties and abdominal pain may be present. Infants who are placed in the prone or left lateral position have been shown to experience significantly less reflux than infants nursed on their backs (Orenstein & Whittington 1983). Although a welcome finding for parents, nurses and infants, there is a wider body of research providing evidence that prone or left lateral positioning in infants is a risk factor for sudden infant death syndrome (Kumar & Sarvanathan 2001). Such evidence needs to be taken into consideration if parents are to be offered sensible, safe advice. Similarly, the results and conclusions of one study need to be considered in the light of other similar studies, as they may differ markedly, depending on the nature of the study design and sample. An oft-quoted example is that of corticosteroids given to women expected to deliver prematurely. A number of individual trials did not identify clear-cut benefits to the treatment; however, when data from all trials were combined in a meta-analysis (see Chapter 7), it became clear that corticosteroids are effective in reducing the risk of death in babies born prematurely (Mulrow 1995).

A wide range of evidence bases relevant to nursing practice

We have mentioned several times that because of the range of settings and people with which nurses work, the concept of EBP is particularly challenging for nurses. Nursing care needs to draw on a wide range of evidence bases, within and beyond the 'medical' sciences, including behavioural and social sciences. In assessing these different kinds of evidence, it is important that nurses can appraise the quality of the research critically, and are able to respect and assess different methodologies.

Public health interventions

Nurses working in public health need to be aware of the evidence about effective interventions in other spheres which can have a beneficial impact on health. A recent review drew together the evidence from trials of effective non-health care interventions which had a beneficial impact on the health of local populations (NHS CRD and UK Cochrane Centre, 1998). Perhaps the best such example is the introduction of legislation to make the wearing of seatbelts compulsory, based on epidemiological evidence of reductions in mortality. There is emerging evidence of the reduction in mortality from road traffic accidents as a result of traffic calming schemes and good evidence that the use of smoke detectors and thermostat controls for tap water can reduce the risk of home injuries (NHS CRD 1996). Nurses working in public health roles, including health visiting, may be in a key position to advocate such schemes.

Health-related behaviours

The example of smoking illustrates why nurses need to be able to draw on evidence from a range of domains of knowledge to inform their work. Smoking is the UK's single greatest cause of preventable illness and death, with more than 120 000 people per year dying from smoking. There is compelling evidence of the health risks associated with direct and passive smoking (Department of Health 1998a). Smoking cessation strategies are therefore a key aspect of current health policy, with investment in smoking cessation clinics in primary care totalling £60 million over 3 years (Figure 1.2). Smoking hits poorer people harder, widening inequalities in health among social groups. To be effective in reducing smoking rates, nurses working with local communities need to understand the role that smoking plays in some people's lives, and why it is that some people smoke although fully cognisant of the

Figure 1.2 **Health authorities, health promotion specialists, education authorities and the news media use posters produced by organisations such as GASP Smoke Free Solutions to discourage smoking. Reproduced with permission from GASP, http://www.gasp.org.uk/gasp.htm**

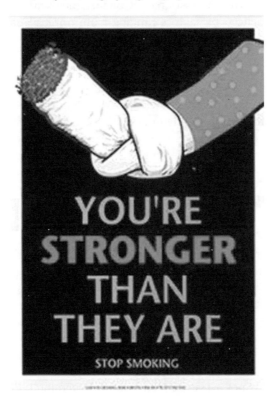

health risks to them and their families. Detailed qualitative work with lone mothers living in poverty illuminated the 'protective' role which smoking played in enabling mothers to cope in very difficult circumstances (Graham 1987, 1988): they balanced smoking's long-term risks against its short-term benefits in enabling them to alleviate the day-to-day stress and flashpoints of caring for young children on very low incomes. The crucial point from this is that any evidence-based anti-smoking strategies must consider alternative supports which would need to be in place to enable such mothers to cope without smoking: to do so would be to truly encapsulate the 'patients' perspectives' as espoused by Sackett et al (2000) as a key dimension of EBM.

Nursing care interventions

In making decisions about interventions (such as drug and other therapies, observations, investigations, etc.), nurses will draw on evidence from multiple sources. Concordance with drug therapy can be influenced by factors ranging from unpleasant side effects of the drug to issues such as perceived recovery from illness, or a denial of the illness or its significance (Beers & Berkow 1999). The approach to the problem of poor concordance with treatment therefore requires knowledge from the psychosocial domain, as well as pharmacological knowledge. Where nurses are required to make decisions about costly interventions such as the use of air fluidised beds (see Chapter 2), or establishing a new post, they will no doubt be obliged to present evidence on the financial costs as well as the increased clinical effectiveness compared with other methods (cost effectiveness) to the management team, as well as details of the clinical efficacy of the intervention.

Communication

We have already argued that nursing care is more than a set of investigations and treatment interventions. As for other professionals, effective communication with communities, clients and patients is a key aspect of high-quality nursing care. Again, this means drawing on a range of bodies of knowledge traditionally conceived of as being outside 'nursing', including communication studies and psychology. Indeed, well-intentioned efforts to implement evidence-based practice may be thwarted and subverted if effective communication is not a feature of the clinical encounter. Psychological research has shown that on receiving bad news there is a limited amount of information that recipients can retain from the first conversation. It is crucial that nurses understand this, so that they do not overload people when they have bad news to give, they keep their first message simple and focused on the key points they need to impart, and they understand the need for on-going support and repeated conversations to enable information to be given at a pace with which recipients can cope.

Management evidence

As nursing roles develop, in the context of a greater emphasis on inter-professional teams in all settings, many will find themselves managing teams, which in some cases may include professions who have traditionally thought of themselves as of higher status than nurses. Again, there is a wide evidence base within management sciences on which nurses can draw to make themselves more effective in those roles. Because of the complexity of organisations and of management (including change management) the research methods employed in management sciences are often more qualitative than those employed in the study of highly focused clinical interventions. The research task is often to understand the organisation and how change is perceived, as much as to study the effectiveness of a complex process of change. Compared with the wealth of research evidence on clinical interventions, organisational change and management issues in the NHS are under-researched (Iles & Sutherland 2001). A new national NHS R&D Programme on Service Delivery and Organisation (SDO) has been set up to fill the yawning gap in organisational and management research in the health sector.

The problem of generalisability

One of the concerns often cited by critics of EBM (as they understand it) relates to the perceived generalisability of published research studies. There are clear dangers with this critique. If proponents really argue that unless the evidence was gathered 'here' it is not relevant, it may be a smoke screen to avoid changing practice. However, it is important that the research undertaken has credibility with its potential users: study population samples need to reflect the composition of target populations for the intervention, the settings and context in which the research is undertaken need to be as 'real life' as possible. In short, it is vital that evidence-based practice is able to draw on practice-based evidence (Hogue 2001, personal communication). For a long time, concerns have been expressed that the distance between academic nursing and the clinical arena has resulted in research that does not relate to the 'reality' of everyday nursing practice (Pearson 2000). Indeed, the key question of how best to generate the evidence base for nursing and ensure its implementation has been around for a long time (Department of Health 1993, 1994, 1995, 1996, 1998b). We all know the perils of developing a research base which is divorced from everyday professional practice. Doctors have wisely avoided that separation, although the combination of academic and professional practice is not without its challenges (Richards 1997).

A study of nursing research outputs between 1988 and 1995 found that although the topics addressed were wide ranging, research concerned with issues relating to the nursing profession (e.g. theory, models, education, research methods, etc.) grew far more rapidly and appeared to be more highly valued than research relating to the care of patients (Traynor et al 2001). The authors postulate that the lower costs and time commitments associated with the former type of research studies, together with the desire to 'self-define' the profession of nursing, may in part account for this difference. This trend in research, of prioritising professional issues over patient care issues, has important ramifications for nurses trying to make informed decisions about aspects of clinical care, particularly with the current and long overdue emphasis given to the patient experience.

When will we get there?

We have demonstrated that the concept of evidence-based practice is not new, but it is reassuring that the commitment to the concept is so firmly stated in recent policies. It is over 30 years since the first academic departments of nursing were established in the UK, and there has been a phenomenal achievement in terms of nursing's integration (and retention) into higher education. But to what extent have we ensured that vibrant R&D activity around nursing issues and perspectives (whether or not it is undertaken by nurses) is really embedded in nursing practice, and the results implemented?

A number of strategies have been implemented and some are starting to pay dividends. For example, Nursing Development Units (NDU) were set up as 'hot-houses for innovation and change in nursing practice' (Redfern et al 1997). The staff of these units are ideally placed to take a leading role in establishing evidence-based practice for nursing; in addition several of the units have been awarded research grants. Urinary catheterisation is just one topic that has been explored in the light of Sackett and colleagues' (1997) definition of evidence-based practice and the organisational infrastructure required for achieving desired outcomes (Adams & Cooke 1998).

The benchmarking process outlined in *The Essence of Care* (Department of Health 2001c) is another development that has the potential to increase an evidence-based approach to nursing care. Different types of evidence have been used to establish benchmark standards which can be used as a starting point for comparing practice, identifying optimum practice and seeking methods to remedy poor practice. The benchmarks are relatively new at the time of writing so have not yet been evaluated, but they are being given a high profile within the UK.

So what else do we need to do to achieve the shift required to make the vision of evidence-based nursing a reality? Some would argue that it is all a matter of money, of ring-fenced budgets for nursing research and research capacity development, to create a safe haven for nurses to develop their skills and evidence base without the risk of medical domination. Certainly profession-specific funding schemes have made a difference and are a necessary component, but they are insufficient to fulfil what is required.

In terms of developing a cadre of nurse researchers, there are key issues concerning the availability of career paths that enable a combination of research and everyday practice; organisational culture and management support for the research ethos in clinical areas; and colleagues' disdain or downright jealousy for the research role as they witness it. For example, the potential profile of nurses' involvement in R&D is not enhanced by the experience of some research nurses, employed on short-term contracts, collecting data for medical colleagues in clinical trials, but without any tangible development of personal research potential, or acknowledgement in publications (Department of Health 1998b).

The welcome commitment in *Making a Difference* (Department of Health 1999) to leadership and R&D within the nursing, midwifery and health visiting professions surely presents us with a golden opportunity. We now need to get on with it, and work to ensure that the next generation of nurses, and those from previous generations who stay (or return) take it for granted that they should seek out and appraise research findings and apply them. This is not always easy, but we owe it to the public to apply our imagination and enthusiasm to make sure that the care they receive is based on the best available evidence.

Acknowledgement

We give special thanks to Aislinn O'Dwyer (Senior Research Fellow, University of Liverpool) for her valuable contribution.

References

Adams F, Cooke M 1998 Implementing evidence-based practice for urinary catheterisation. British Journal of Nursing 7(22): 1393–1399

Beers MH and Berkow R (eds) 1999 Merck manual of diagnosis and therapy, 17th edition. Section 22, Clinical pharmacology, Chapter 301, Factors affecting drug response. NJ: Merck Research Laboratories

Bury TJ, Mead JM (eds) 1998 Evidence-based healthcare: a practical guide for therapists. Oxford: Butterworth-Heinemann

Cullum N, Nelson E, Fletcher A, Sheldon T 2001 Compression for venous leg ulcers (Cochrane Review). In: The Cochrane Library, Disk Issue 2, 2001. Oxford: Update Software

Department of Health 1993 Report of the task force on the strategy for research in nursing, midwifery and health visiting. London: Department of Health

Department of Health 1994 Supporting research and development in the NHS: report of the R&D task force (The Culyer Report). London: Department of Health

Department of Health 1995 A research workforce strategy. Paper to Central Research and Development Committee, July 1995 (CRDCP95-22). London: Department of Health

Department of Health 1996 Research capacity strategy for the Department of Health and the NHS. A first statement. London: Department of Health

Department of Health 1997 The new NHS: modern and dependable. London: Department of Health

Department of Health 1998a Smoking kills. London: Department of Health

Department of Health 1998b Developing human resources for health related R&D: next steps. Report of the R&D workforce capacity development group (The Pearson Report). London: Department of Health

Department of Health 1999 Making a difference: strengthening the nursing, midwifery and health visiting contribution to health and health care. London: Department of Health

Department of Health 2000a Towards a strategy for nursing research and development: proposals for action. London: Department of Health

Department of Health 2000b The NHS plan: a plan for investment. A plan for reform. London: Department of Health

Department of Health 2001a Standard principles for preventing hospital acquired infections. Journal of Hospital Infection 47 (Supplement): S21–S37

Department of Health 2001b Working together – Learning together: A framework for lifelong learning for the NHS. London: Department of Health

Department of Health 2001c The essence of care: patient-focused benchmarking for health care practitioners. http://www.doh.gov.uk/essenceofcare/essenceofcare

Fibrinolytic Therapy Trialists (FTT) Collaborative Group 1994 Indications for fibrinolytic therapy in suspected acute myocardial infarction: collaborative overview of early mortality and major morbidity results from all randomised trials of over 1000 patients. Lancet 343: 311–322

Graham H 1987 Women's smoking and family health. Social Science and Medicine 25: 47–56

Graham H 1988 Women and smoking in the United Kingdom: implications for health promotion. Health Promotion Journal 3(4): 371–382

Grahame Smith D 1998 Evidence based medicine: challenging the authority. Journal of the Royal Society of Medicine (Suppl 35): 7–11

Handwashing Liaison Group 1999 Hand washing. A modest measure – with big effects. Editorial. British Medical Journal 318: 686

Harrison JE 2000 Evidence-based orthodontics – how do I assess the evidence? Journal of Orthodontics 27(2): 189–197

Iles V, Sutherland K 2001 Organisational change: a review for health care managers, professionals and researchers. London: NCCSDO, London School of Hygiene and Tropical Medicine

Kumar Y, Sarvanathan R 2001 Gastro-oesophageal reflux in children. In: Clinical evidence, Issue 5. London: BMJ Publishing Group, pp 253–259

Lewith GT 1996 The use and abuse of evidence-based medicine: an example from general practice. In: Ernst E (ed.) Complementary medicine: an objective appraisal. Oxford: Butterworth-Heinemann

Muir Gray JA 1997 Evidence-based health care: how to make health policy and management decisions. New York: Churchill Livingstone

Mulrow CD 1995 Rationale for systematic reviews. In: Chalmers I, Altman DG (eds) Systematic reviews. London: BMJ Publishing Group, p 1.

NHS CRD (NHS Centre for Reviews and Dissemination) 1996 Preventing unintentional injuries in children and young adolescents. Effective Health Care 2(5)

NHS CRD and UK Cochrane Centre 1998 Evidence from systematic reviews of research relevant to the forthcoming White Paper on Public Health. Oxford: UK Cochrane Centre

Orenstein SR, Whitington PF 1983 Positioning for prevention of infant gastro-oesophageal reflux. Journal of Pediatrics 103: 534–537

Pearson M 2000 Making a difference through research: how nurses can turn the vision into reality (editorial). NT Research 5(2): 85–86

Plowman R, Graves N, Griffin M, Roberts J, Swan T, Cookson B, Taylor L 1999 The socio-economic burden of hospital-acquired infection. London: Public Health Laboratory Service

Plowman R, Graves N, Griffin M, Roberts J, Swan T, Cookson B, Taylor L 2001 The rate and cost of hospital acquired infections occurring in patients admitted to selected specialties of a district general hospital in England and the national burden imposed. Journal of Hospital Infection 47(3): 198–209

Pursey A, Quinney D, Pearson M 1997 Concepts of care in primary health care nursing. In: Hugman R, Peelo M, Soothill K (eds) Concepts of care. London: Edward Arnold

Redfern S, Norman I, Murrells T, Christian S, Gilmore A et al 1997 External review of the Department of Health-funded nursing development units. Executive Summary. Available from Nursing Research Unit, King's College London, Cornwall House, Waterloo Road, London SE1 8WA

Richards R 1997 Clinical academic careers: report of an independent task force. London: Wellcome Trust.

Rotter ML 1997 150 years of hand disinfection. Semmelweis' heritage. Hygiene and Medizin 22: 332–339

Sackett D, Richardson WS, Rosenberg W, Haynes RB 1997 Evidence based medicine: how to practice and teach EBM. New York: Churchill Livingstone

Sackett DL, Strauss SE, Richardson WS, Rosenberg W, Haynes RB 2000 Evidence-Based Medicine. How to Practice and Teach EBM 2nd edn. London: Churchill Livingstone

Traynor M, Rafferty AM, Lewison G 2001 Endogenous and exogenous research? Findings from a bibliometric study of UK nursing research. Journal of Advanced Nursing 34(2): 212–222

Tully MP, Cantrill J 1999 Role of the pharmacist in evidence-based prescribing in primary care. In: Gabbay M (ed.) The evidence-based primary care handbook. London: Royal Society of Medicine, pp 183–193

Wellcome Trust 2001 Putting NHS research on the map: an analysis of scientific publications in England, 1990–97. London: The Wellcome Trust Publishing Department

Section 2

SKILLS FOR EVIDENCE-BASED PRACTICE

2

How to ask the right question

Jean V Craig

Key points

■ Clinical decisions need to take account of current best evidence
■ The process of achieving this entails a number of steps
■ A starting point is to formulate a clearly defined question. The question drives each step of the process and should therefore be carefully considered at the outset
■ A well formulated question maximises the potential of finding relevant evidence that can be applied to a specific patient in a specific setting.

Introduction

The process for ensuring that clinical decisions are, as far as possible, informed by current research evidence has been described by Sackett et al (2000). This five-step approach entails:

1. Converting information needs into clear questions
2. Seeking evidence to answer those questions
3. Evaluating (critically appraising) the evidence for its validity (truthfulness) and usefulness
4. Integrating findings with clinical expertise, patient needs, patient preferences and, if appropriate, applying these findings
5. Evaluating performance (and the outcome of our decision/practice).

This approach is driven by the belief that up-to-date research findings, when used to inform clinical decisions, may increase the likelihood that required outcomes are achieved. This chapter focuses on the first step: converting information needs into focused questions. A carefully formulated question maximises the likelihood that relevant, high-quality evidence is identified and incorporated appropriately into the decision-making process. Information needs are not always clear-cut. This can result in hours of non-focused reading of literature that may or may not be relevant or applicable. A strategy for developing 'answerable' clinical questions is therefore invaluable to health care professionals who aim to integrate best evidence, clinical expertise and patient preferences and values in reaching decisions (Sackett et al 2000).

Decision-making in clinical practice

Nurses and other health care practitioners make numerous decisions when caring for their patients. Consider the range of activities carried out during the course of a morning by a nurse working in a general practice. These could include:

- syringing the ears of a patient complaining of wax build-up
- discussing asthma preventative measures with a concerned mother
- performing a cervical smear test
- advising a patient with acute lower back pain
- immunising an infant
- running a clinic for patients with Type 2 (non-insulin-dependent diabetes mellitus).

The decisions relating to each of these interventions are diverse and multiple. For example, where a patient presents with decreased hearing in one ear caused by a build-up of wax, the nurse must decide on the most appropriate treatment. Ear syringing is not without risk. Otitis externa, damage to the external auditory canal, perforation of the tympanic membrane, pain and vertigo have all been reported (Sharp et al 1990). Modern, electronic pulsed syringes are available, but metal syringes, for which the rate of irrigation has to be manually controlled, are still used in some practices (Stubbs 2001). In patients with previous tympanic membrane perforation or grommets, the risk of complications may be increased. In a review by the Medical Defence Union (MDU), ear syringing was shown to account for 19% of claims involving general practice procedures. Complications were related to poor technique, faulty equipment, exertion of excess pressure, and failure to examine the ear (Price 1997). In more than half of the claims it was the practice nurse who performed the procedure. The MDU review helps to highlight the importance of informed decision-making. The nurse, together with the patient, will need to consider the potential effectiveness and potential risks of the procedure, before proceeding. Less immediate but equally important decisions will need to be addressed: Should equipment be updated? What training is needed? Is a competency testing programme required?

The practice nurse will need to make numerous other decisions during the course of the morning. For example, advice on the prevention of acute asthma will entail decisions about possible trigger factors, likelihood of compliance with specific treatment, methods for administering the treatment, effectiveness of the treatment, methods for educating the child and family, etc. For infant immunisation the nurse must decide what information a parent needs in order to make a well-informed choice.

In making the above decisions, the nurse will be influenced (consciously or unconsciously) by a number of factors (Box 2.1). Each of these factors plays an important role in decision-making, but when used in isolation may result in inappropriate decisions. The application of scientific evidence without considered judgement results in a 'cook book' approach to health care, with nurses slavishly following recipes for care, regardless of the patient's specific needs. In contrast, over-reliance on personal experience when making decisions can be equally damaging. For example, if practice nurses continue to recommend bed rest to people with acute lower back pain because it appears to have worked in the past, they will be ignoring recent evidence that bed rest may impair rehabilitation (Hagen et al 2000). In people with type 2 (non-insulin dependent) diabetes mellitus, one-off routine annual testing of urine may be the usual practice, however recent evidence indicates that a single annual near-patient test is not sufficiently sensitive in identifying people with renal disease. Instead urine should be tested at least annually and on more than one occasion for proteinuria and, if found to be negative, it should subsequently be tested for microalbuminuria (NHS CRD 2000).

Up-to-date, valid evidence, directly relevant to the situation at hand, needs to be integrated together with the other influencing factors in order to maximise the likelihood of the expected out-

Box 2.1   Factors influencing the decision-making process

- Up-to-date research evidence
- Clinical expertise:
  - formal education
  - accumulated knowledge (journal articles, text books, press reports, expert opinion, advice from colleagues, clinical audit)
  - past experience, built on a case-by-case basis
  - most recent experience
  - skill level
- Beliefs, attitudes, values, tradition
- Routine, 'the way things are done around here'
- Factors relating to the patient and their family:
  - clinical circumstances, co-morbid conditions
  - preferences, values, beliefs, attitudes, expectations, concerns
  - needs
- Organisational factors
  - national and local policies
  - service/resource availability
  - funding
  - equipment
  - time

come being achieved. In the course of one morning, our practice nurse identifies a number of information needs, arising from interactions with his or her patients. Examples of these information needs are presented in Box 2.2. These questions have been phrased in a general way, and are therefore not easily answerable. If the practice nurse is to be successful in making an evidence-based decision, the questions will need to be much more focused.

Turning information needs into focused questions

There is an art to phrasing questions in such a way as to elicit a meaningful answer, whether these are questions that are directed at people, or questions asked of the literature.

Box 2.2 Examples of information needs

- What treatment should I offer to this patient with wax build-up in the ear?
- Should our practice purchase an electronic ear syringe?
- How can we (practice nurse, child, family, doctor) prevent further acute asthma episodes in this child?
- How can I persuade this child to take his asthma treatments regularly?
- What advice should I give to this person with back pain?
- Do cervical smear tests with normal results accurately exclude cervical cancer?
- Should we be testing for chlamydia at the time of cervical smear?
- What is the best way of monitoring for complications of diabetes?

As with the research process, the evidence-based process flows from the question. In research, the study design and methods are determined by what it is the researcher wants to know. It is by continuously refining the question that the researcher decides on the study design, the research methods, the sample population, the intervention (if any), and the outcomes of interest. Similarly, in an approach that aims to incorporate best evidence in decision-making, it is the clinical question that drives each of the subsequent steps. There are three key reasons for focusing questions: (i) facilitating the search for relevant evidence, (ii) sorting best evidence from weaker, less valid evidence, and (iii) deciding whether the evidence is applicable to our patients. (These three areas are dealt with in detail in Chapters 3, 4 and 5 respectively.)

(i) Searching for evidence

The more explicit the question, the easier it is to run searches on electronic databases such as those contained within the Cochrane Library, CINAHL (Cumulative Index of Allied Health and Nursing Literature), or MEDLINE. The key components of the question are used to devise a methodical search strategy that aims to yield a manageable number of relevant research studies. A non-focused question is more likely to yield larger numbers of non-relevant studies than a focused question, and valuable search time will be wasted trying to sift through the long list of retrieved references for relevant studies. For example, the practice nurse wants to know what advice to give to a patient with back pain and decides to search the MEDLINE database by using the phrase 'back pain'. Searching MEDLINE from 1966 to June 2001 yields 4994 references. Even when limiting the search to the last 2 years, 2270 references are retrieved, many of which relate to pregnancy and child birth and are therefore unlikely to be of relevance to her male patient. A focused question will help to overcome this problem by providing guidance to the search strategy.

(ii) Selecting the best evidence

Once the question has been formulated, the type of study design that should be used to answer that question can be identified (Logan & Gilbert 2000). For example, a question about the effectiveness of a treatment is best addressed by a well-conducted systematic review of randomised controlled trials or by a randomised controlled trial. For a question relating to non-compliance with a treatment, the best evidence would be a well-conducted qualitative study. Where information about the prognosis of a disease is required, the best evidence would be provided by a good-quality cohort study. A search of electronic databases may yield a large number of research studies that appear to be relevant to the clinical question. Knowing which type of study design would best answer the question enables rapid sorting of the retrieved studies into a 'hierarchy', such that studies with the most appropriate study design take precedence. Studies lower down the hierarchy need only be consulted where there is a lack of better quality evidence. It is worth remembering, however, that less than optimal study designs may have to be used. For example, it may be impractical, unethical, or impossible to carry out a randomised controlled trial when assessing the adverse effects or effectiveness of certain interventions (e.g. in a study looking at the adverse effects of smoking, it is not possible to randomise participants to the intervention or the control group). Further information about study designs is given in Chapter 4.

(iii) Applying the evidence

When a well-conducted study has been located, a judgement has to be made as to the likelihood of the results from the research being achieved if they were applied to a specific patient. It is unlikely that the circumstances in which the research study was undertaken will exactly match the clinical situation. Nurses reading a research study must therefore decide whether the participants in the study are so dissimilar from their patient that the results cannot be applied to their situation. For example, is it appropriate to apply the results of a study that looked at methods for improving compliance with drug treatment in the elderly, to a population of teenagers? Methods that are effective in the elderly, such as the dispensing of tablets into individual containers labelled with the days of the week, may be seen by adolescents as embarrassing and may in fact result in reduced compliance. Similarly, a judgement must be made as to whether a similar, but not identical, intervention or test will be likely to bring about the same result as that achieved in the study. A carefully formulated question includes a description of the patient group of interest, the planned treatment or investigation, and the key outcomes that the patient hopes to achieve. It is therefore a useful tool for screening out those research studies that are not applicable to the clinical situation, or for helping to ensure that differences between the patient and the research population are transparent.

A framework for formulating questions

The PICO (population, intervention, comparison intervention, outcome) framework, devised by Sackett et al (1997), is a useful method for making questions more focused. The question is built in four (or three) parts (Box 2.3). Careful thought is required when deciding how general or how specific each part of the question should be. For population, it may be necessary to specify age, gender, disease type, disease severity or co-morbidity. This will depend on whether the results of a very broad, inclusive population could be applied to your specific patient group. The intervention (or test or exposure) may need to be described in some detail to ensure clarity. This is especially important for multi-faceted interventions (such as asthma clinics, nurse development units, etc.) where any number of factors may be responsible for the outcome of interest.

Box 2.3 The four (or three)-part question (PICO)

Patient or problem: Define who or what the question is about
Tip: describe a group of patients similar to yours

Intervention: Define which intervention, test or exposure you are interested in
An intervention is a planned course of action. An exposure is something that happens such as a fall, anxiety, exposure to house dust mites, etc. (Bury & Mead 1998)
Tip: describe what it is you are considering doing or what it is that has happened to the patient

Comparison intervention (if any):   Define the alternate intervention
Tip: describe the alternative that can be compared with the intervention

Outcomes: Define the important outcomes, beneficial or harmful
Tip: Define what you are hoping to achieve or avoid

Deciding on the most important outcomes is not always straight-forward, but can be facilitated by considering the patient's perspective. Very general outcomes may be difficult to measure, and details of how outcomes can be objectively measured may need to be specified.

The formula cannot always be easily applied, but nevertheless it is a useful tool. The scenarios below illustrate the use of this formula.

Case study 2.1

A 10-year-old girl who has had open-heart surgery has been very ill for 2 days, requiring artificial ventilation and a number of support drugs to maintain her blood pressure. The little girl has developed a small pressure sore at the back of her head.

The nurse asks the following question:

> How can I prevent further pressure sores from developing in this child?

This general question may be difficult to answer. Many factors contribute to tissue breakdown, including poor nutrition, poor circulation, immobility, and type of mattress. The nurse decides to focus on the mattress. The child is currently being nursed on a high specification foam mattress.

At this stage it is important to invest time in further refining the question. This will yield dividends when the nurse comes to search for relevant research studies. Each component of the question must be carefully considered:

Population

The nurse must ask herself whether research carried out in the adult population could be applied to children. The decision of whether to exclude specific age groups is usually based on the known differences in the response to disease, treatments, and tests, by each age group, or on the inferred differences which might arise from the above. If the differences are such that the results of a research study will not be generalisable from one age group to another, then age groups need to be defined within the question.

In addition, it is important to consider whether, and how specifically, to define the condition. Is there any reason for restricting the question to patients who have had cardiac surgery? Critically ill cardiac patients may have poor circulation, and therefore be at increased risk of developing pressure sores, however other groups of critically ill children (for example children with septicaemia) may also have poor perfusion. One could argue that all critically ill children are probably at similar risk of developing pressure sores, and research carried out in these patients, regardless of their diagnosis, would no doubt help to answer the question.

Intervention (or test or exposure)

A variety of mattresses and beds are available on the market, ranging from standard hospital foam or high specification foam, to constant low-pressure devices or alternating pressure devices. Some of these devices may be more effective than others. Depending on the device under consideration, there could be major cost implications. In the year 2000, costs of pressure-relieving devices were found to range from £100 to £30 000 (Cullum et al 2000). The nurse does not want to be so specific with the question as to limit the chance of finding any relevant evidence, but by clarifying what pressure-relieving device she plans to use for the 10-year-old patient (we will assume this to be the constant low-pressure bed), the search for information is made easier.

Comparison intervention

It is not always necessary to define a comparison intervention, but in this case, the intervention against which the proposed device could be compared is the method currently in use. Let us suppose this is the high-specification foam mattress.

Outcome

Outcomes may need to be carefully defined. The nurse wants to prevent further pressure sores. By this she may mean the prevention of persistent discolouration or/and breakdown of the skin. Research studies that define pressure sores as 'partial or full thickness skin loss', may have different results to research studies that include in their definition 'persistent discolouration of the skin'.

In summary:

- *Population*:   Critically ill children
- *Intervention*: Constant low-pressure beds
- *Comparison*: High specification foam mattresses
- *Outcome*:   Pressure sores: constant discolouration of skin, or partial or full thickness skin loss.

Our more focused question could therefore be:

> In critically ill children, are constant low-pressure beds more effective than high specification foam mattresses in preventing pressure sores (defined here as constant discolouration of the skin, or partial or full thickness skin loss)?

At this stage it is useful to identify which type of study design is most likely to provide a valid (believable) answer to the question. As this is a question about effectiveness of a therapy, the study design of choice is a systematic review of randomised controlled trials or a randomised controlled trial. Retrieved studies can be sorted accordingly, with studies of the above design being given highest priority.

Searching for research evidence is covered in detail in Chapter 3, but it is worth briefly mentioning here that all four parts of the question are not always used when developing a search strategy. The nurse could run a preliminary search using terms relating to the *population* (for example 'child', 'paediatric', etc.) and *intervention* (for example 'low-pressure bed') parts of the question. If this resulted in thousands of hits (references), terms relating to the *comparison intervention* or even the *outcome* could also be added. This should further restrict the number of hits and enhance the likelihood of the references being relevant to the question.

The nurse will be able to check the retrieved articles against the focused question. Those that are found to be less applicable (for example, studies that have focused on adults that are obese) can be set aside in favour of the more applicable studies, i.e. the studies that are generalisable to the 10-year-old child.

We have looked at one question in detail, but the nurse may have a number of information needs relating to this patient. Some of the questions arising from these information needs are highlighted in Table 2.1.

Case study 2.2

Alison, a 2-year-old infant, presented at the local accident and emergency department with fever and vomiting. In line with departmental policy, urine was collected in a bag (which had been applied to her perineum according to the manufacturer's instructions), then sent for microscopy and culture. The white cell count was found to be high and Alison was started on a course of antibiotics. When she returned for follow-up 5 days later, the attending physician was frustrated to note that the culture results showed a mixed growth. It was not clear whether Alison had indeed suffered a urinary tract infection (UTI), or whether the urine sample had simply been contaminated. In view of the risk of underlying urinary tract abnormalities and potential upper urinary tract damage, children with UTI need to be investigated carefully. The physician, concerned that the methods used for obtaining urine samples are inappropriate, suggests that bag-catch urine sampling should be abandoned in favour of clean-catch urine sampling. This

Table 2.1 Other questions about prevention or treatment of pressure sores

Population or problem	Intervention (or test or exposure)	Comparison intervention (if any)	Outcome
Patients with pressure sores (partial or full thickness skin loss)	Application of hydrocolloids	Application of gauze dressings	Reduced time to healing Faster shrinkage of the pressure sore
Patients with pressure sores (partial or full thickness skin loss)	Ascorbic acid supplementation	Usual diet with no additional supplements	Reduced time to healing Faster shrinkage of the pressure sore
Critically ill children	Constant low-pressure devices, or alternating pressure devices	Three hourly lifting or turning	Prevention of pressure sores, defined here as discolouration of the skin, or partial or full thickness skin loss Risk of destabilising the patient, poor cardiac output Costs

entails catching a spontaneously voided urine. The infant's nappy is removed and their carer is provided with a sterile container and instructed to watch for the opportunity to catch the urine. The nurses on the unit are worried about the implications of changing practice. They feel that this method is more likely to cause delays for patients and their families.

They want to know:

> What is the best way of obtaining a urine specimen for culture, from a child?

We can check how focused the question is, by examining each component individually.

Population

The population of interest is children suspected of having UTI, however the nurses may want to consider further defining the population.

The results of a study carried out in older children (who may be able to obtain the urine specimen themselves) are likely to be different to those from a study carried out in children still wearing nappies.

Intervention (or test or exposure)

In this case, the existing method of urine sampling is by urine bag. It may be useful to include brief details as to the methods involved in obtaining bag-catch urine specimens as these may differ from those used by researchers and this could affect the results.

Comparison intervention

Comparing two methods is a useful way of reaching a decision about a practice change. Where the topic of interest is a diagnostic test, the method should be compared against a reference standard, which in this case is supra-pubic aspiration of urine directly from the bladder. There can be disadvantages to using reference standard methods: supra-pubic aspiration is more difficult to perform, more invasive, and more painful than either the bag-catch or clean-catch method.

Outcome

The key outcome of interest is whether the method results in contamination of the culture specimen. Other outcomes that the nurses may wish to consider are time, acceptability to patient and family and ease of use.

In summary:

- *Population*: Children suspected of having UTI, who are not yet toilet trained
- *Intervention*: Bag-catch urine specimens
- *Comparison*: Supra-pubic aspiration
- *Outcome*: False positive culture contamination.

The revised question is:

> In children suspected of having UTI, who are not yet toilet trained, is the risk of false positive culture contamination greater when urine is obtained by bag-catch, as compared with urine obtained by supra-pubic aspiration directly from the bladder?

In addition to establishing the risk of culture contamination by urine-bag sampling, the nurses need to establish the risk for clean-catch urine sampling (examples of additional questions are given in Table 2.2).

Table 2.2 Other questions about diagnosis of urinary tract infection

Population or problem	Intervention (or test or exposure)	Comparison intervention (if any)	Outcome
Children suspected of having UTI, who are not yet toilet trained	Clean-catch urine sampling using a sterile container	Supra-pubic aspiration directly from bladder	False positive culture contamination
Obtaining urine samples from children who are not yet toilet trained	Clean-catch method	Bag-catch method	Time taken to successfully obtain urine sample Cost Parent satisfaction Nurse satisfaction

Case study 2.3

A recent public health report shows that despite national initiatives to promote breast feeding, uptake is poor. A health visitor who works in a deprived, inner city community and visits mothers from day 10 after delivery has noticed that many of the mothers feed their babies with infant milk formula rather than breast milk. The health visitor wants to gain a better understanding of the factors that influence mothers to bottle feed with infant milk formula. This information may help to inform future educational programmes aimed at promoting breast feeding.

The health visitor asks:

Why do mothers not breastfeed?

The question does not easily fit the PICO formula, but it is nevertheless useful to consider each component of the question. It may be possible to further refine the question, thereby improving the chance of finding relevant research evidence.

Population

The educational programme will be aimed at mothers who live in a deprived area of the city, a population that has different needs and different experiences to women in less deprived areas. In this case, the health visitor is interested in the views of mothers of all ages, however, if the problem were specific to very young, first-time mothers, the question would need to reflect this. The health visitor may find it useful to examine the views of both breastfeeding and bottlefeeding mothers in order to obtain information about the factors that influence mothers in their decision to breast or bottle feed.

Intervention (or test or exposure)

Unlike questions relating to test accuracy, or effectiveness of a treatment, there is no intervention for this type of question. The health visitor is interested in gaining insight into factors that influence the mothers' decisions. Once these factors have been established, the health visitor can start to develop a programme of interventions to promote breast feeding.

Outcomes

The health visitor is interested in mothers' perceptions, attitudes, values or beliefs relating to breast feeding and/or to bottle feeding with infant formula.

The revised question is as follows:

> What are the factors identified by mothers who live in deprived inner city areas that influence them to breast feed or to bottle feed using infant milk formula?

The type of research that is most likely to provide an in-depth understanding of the views of the mothers is qualitative research (discussed in Chapter 6).

Becoming proficient in asking questions

Asking the right question is a skill that requires practice. The following exercises are a useful starting point for practising this skill but are no substitute for the real-life problems that are encountered in day-to-day practice. To become adept at this skill, nurses will need to practise translating real-life information needs into focused questions on a daily basis.

Exercises

Try to formulate focused questions from the following scenarios. You may want to think about the study design that is most likely to provide valid results for each of the questions (study design is addressed fully in Chapter 4). Some suggestions for focused questions that might arise from these scenarios are given in Appendix 2.1 (page 43).

Exercise 2.1

Mrs York, a 52-year-old woman, sustained a severe wrist fracture following a fall. She was subsequently investigated for, and found to have, osteoporosis. Her doctor discussed the potential benefits and harms of hormone replacement therapy (HRT) with her and together they decided that she should start the treatment. Mrs York has since spoken to family and friends about the potential risks of HRT, and has become increasingly concerned that she may be at risk of breast cancer. During a well woman's clinic, she tells the practice nurse that she is thinking of stopping the treatment.

Mrs York is a heavy smoker. Smoking, caffeine and lack of exercise have all been shown to contribute to osteoporosis. The nurse wonders how best to help Mrs York make the required lifestyle changes.

Exercise 2.2

Mrs Hardy, the mother of a young infant, is trying to decide whether to give up smoking. Her infant has recently had episodes of wheezing and breathlessness, requiring admission to hospital for a couple of nights. Mrs Hardy has been warned about the risks of respiratory problems in children who are exposed to cigarette smoke, but she wants to know if there really is a link between the two.

Exercise 2.3

Jennifer is attending general practice for a cervical smear test. She has read in the newspaper that a number of women who underwent cervical smear tests, and had negative test results, were later found to have cervical cancer. Jennifer is very nervous about having any tests at all, and is tempted to cancel the smear test in view of the possibility of the results being inaccurate.

Exercise 2.4

A practice nurse has advised Mr Reynolds, a 60-year-old man who is overweight and has hypertension, to reduce weight and to cut down on the amount of salt in his diet. Mr Reynolds is very sceptical that this course of action will help him. The nurse would like to find some evidence that supports her recommendation.

Specific prompts for accessing research evidence

Health care practitioners should constantly evaluate their practice. New technologies (for example drugs, blood pressure monitoring devices, wound dressings) are introduced on a regular basis; different processes of care (case management, patient-held records, home care of long-term ventilated patients, etc.) are explored; and new information (for example factors associated with sudden infant death syndrome, literacy figures for the adult population, etc.) is published at regular intervals. A questioning approach to health care is important if such 'innovations' are to be identified in the first place and, secondly, if they are to be considered for inclusion in the management of patients. An attitude of 'research mindedness' (Perkins et al 1999, page 4), where questions such as 'Which is best?', 'Who should do this?', 'Where should this patient be treated?' is needed. Blind acceptance of a technology that is skilfully marketed by a company representative, or outright rejection of change to an existing practice, could potentially impact negatively on patient outcome, resources and cost.

Although nurses would agree with the above, the need to access research evidence in the context of the clinical setting is not always apparent. One of the challenges for nurses and other health care professionals is to recognise the importance of asking questions about their practice.

Prompts for consulting scientific evidence include:

- uncertainty as to the best course of action
- controversy regarding the way a procedure or therapy should be carried out
- lack of knowledge about the effectiveness of one therapy or test over another
- unexpected patient outcomes
- the introduction of new therapies or technologies

■ practices based on tradition
■ 'novel' suggestions by patients.

For those aspects of care that are already entrenched in day-to-day practice, a questioning approach is equally important, but perhaps more difficult to achieve. Where a method of care delivery (for example the 'drugs round' where drugs are dispensed to all ward patients, at set times, by a designated nurse) has become accepted as routine practice, practitioners may accept it as the right or only method, and alternatives may not be considered. In addition, 'ritualistic' practices which consume valuable nursing time and resources, and may carry little or no benefit or may even cause harm, must be examined for clinical and cost effectiveness.

It may be helpful for the nurse to consider whether 'the right person, is doing the right thing, in the right way, in the right place, at the right time, with the right result' (Graham 1996). By asking this question, any information gaps will be highlighted. Finally, reflection, a strategy used within nursing to encourage learning from practical experiences (Boud et al 1985), can be used as another method for identifying information needs. By reflecting on 'critical incidents', gaps in knowledge of current research findings can be identified.

Prioritising questions

The volume of decisions and related information needs that arise each day can be overwhelming. It may be necessary to prioritise the questions for which best evidence is to be sought. Questions that are most important to the patient's well-being, that arise repeatedly (Sackett et al 1997) or that have potentially important consequences (such as risk or cost reductions), could be considered high priority questions. At the Evidence Based Child Health Unit in Liverpool, topics are prioritised according to the following criteria:

■ Relevant to the Trust and to NHS priorities
■ Affects a significant number of patients
■ Potential to implement change in practice
■ Demand for the topic from a number of independent sources
■ Wide variations in practice
■ Genuine uncertainty or controversy as to best practice.

Questions for research

In the spirit of evidence-based practice, this chapter has focused on questions that nurses in the clinical field are asking; questions which they hope can be answered to some extent by previously published research evidence. However the same PICO formula can be applied to many research questions (that may or may not arise directly from an interaction with a patient or clinical problem). In research, as with evidence-based practice, the question drives the research project. Asking a general, unfocused question will lead to difficulties at each step of the research process.

Summary

The success or failure of explicitly basing nursing practice on best evidence, relies on nurses challenging both new and established methods of caring for patients. The skills provided in this chapter provide a starting point for seeking out good-quality evidence to support current practice or a change in practice (Box 2.4). This first step in the evidence-based process is an important one and nurses who take the time to develop carefully worded questions will be well rewarded at each stage in the process.

Box 2.4 Quick reference: what to do in clinical practice

- Consider what information is required when making a health care decision.
- Prioritise which information need to address.
- Formulate a question.
- Focus the question using the PICO formula.
- Decide how specific or how general each part of the question needs to be.
- Decide which study design is most likely to provide valid results.
- Refer to the focused question at each stage of the evidence-based process, i.e. when searching for or appraising evidence, and when applying the evidence to your situation.

References

Boud D, Keogh R, Walker D 1985 Reflection: turning experience into learning. London: Kogan Press

Bury TJ, Mead JM (eds) 1998 Evidence based healthcare: a practical guide for therapists. Oxford: Butterworth-Heinemann

Cullum N, Deeks J, Sheldon TA, Song F, Fletcher AW 2000 Beds, mattresses and cushions for pressure sore prevention and treatment (Cochrane Review). In: The Cochrane Library, Issue 3, 2000. Oxford: Update Software

Graham G 1996 Clinically effective medicine in a rational health service. Health Director June 11–12

Hagen K, Hilde G, Jamtvedt G, Winnem M 2000 Bedrest for acute low back pain and sciatica (Cochrane Review). In: The Cochrane Library, Issue 4, 2000. Oxford: Update Software

Logan S, Gilbert R 2000 Framing questions. In: Moyer VA, Elliot EJ, Davis RL, et al (eds) Evidence based paediatrics and child health. London: BMJ Books

NHS CRD (Centre for Reviews and Dissemination) 2000 Complications of diabetes: renal disease and promotion of self-management. Effective Health Care Bulletin 6(1)

Perkins ER, Simnett I, Wright L 1999 Creative tensions in evidence-based practice. In: Perkins ER, Simnett I, Wright L (eds) Evidence based health promotion. New York: Wiley

Price J 1997 Problems of ear syringing. Practice Nurse 14(2): 126–127

Sackett DL, Richardson WS, Rosenberg W, Haynes RB 1997 Evidence based medicine: how to practice and teach EBM. London: Churchill Livingstone

Sackett DL, Strauss SE, Richardson WS, Rosenberg W, Haynes RB 2000 Evidence-based medicine: how to practice and teach EBM, 2nd edn. London: Churchill Livingstone

Sharp JF, Wilson JA, Ross L, Barr-Hamilton RM 1990 Ear wax removal: a survey of current practice. British Medical Journal 301: 1251–1252

Stubbs G 2001 Getting to grips with the metal ear syringe. Nursing Times 97(20): 40

Appendix 2.1
Possible solutions to exercises

Exercise 2.1 – Mrs York

Question 1

Population:	In post-menopausal women with no family history of breast cancer
Intervention (exposure):	how much does hormone replacement therapy
Outcomes:	increase the risk of breast cancer?
Optimal study design:	Cohort study

Question 2

Population:	In post-menopausal women with osteoporosis
Intervention:	does hormone replacement therapy
Comparison:	compared with no hormone replacement therapy
Outcome:	reduce the risk of fractures?
Optimal study design:	Systematic review of randomised controlled trials or randomised controlled trial

Exercise 2.2 – Mrs Hardy and her infant

Population:	In children
Exposure:	who are exposed to passive smoking
Outcome:	what is the risk of respiratory disease?
Optimal study design:	Cohort study

Exercise 2.3 – Jennifer

Population:	In women
Intervention:	who have cervical smear tests
Outcome:	what is the risk of failing to identify cervical cancer in affected women? and what is the risk of falsely identifying cervical cancer in non-affected women?
Optimal study design:	Blinded comparison of test and reference standard test

Exercise 2.4 – Mr Reynolds

Question 1

Population:	In men over 50 years of age who are hypertensive
Intervention:	does a weight-reducing diet (or replace this with 'does limiting dietary salt intake')
Outcome:	lower blood pressure and reduce the risk of stroke and cardiovascular mortality?
Optimal study design:	Systematic review of randomised controlled trials or randomised controlled trial

Question 2

Population:	In middle-aged men who have a health condition related to being overweight (the population has been restricted to middle aged men as their attitudes and perceptions of factors such as body image, their cooking abilities, choice of food etc. may differ from those of younger men)
Intervention:	(there is no intervention in this case)
Outcome:	what are their perceptions/attitudes towards weight reducing diets?
Optimal study design:	Qualitative research

3

Searching the literature

Olwen Beaven

Key points

- Identifying best evidence requires an understanding of basic search principles. More advanced techniques will help to enhance a search
- Systematic reviews require more extensive searching
- The internet can be a valuable source of information, especially if reliable/quality assessed resources are used.

Introduction

The purpose of this chapter is to provide a beginner's guide to the principles and practice of searching the research literature. Whilst it is unrealistic to teach the art of searching within the constraints of the printed page, it is possible to pass on a basic understanding of the search process and the core competencies needed to enable readers to progress and develop their searching skills. Whilst this chapter is primarily aimed at novice searchers, it will be useful revision for those who feel more confident and there are also some sections targeted specifically at the advanced searcher. The importance of searching the literature to find information is often overlooked in the hurry to develop new ideas, try new approaches or to get research underway. However, a good literature search can underpin the whole problem-solving process – if key information is missing, it is much harder to identify an appropriate solution. This is particularly true when searching the research literature to try to answer specific clinical questions.

Where is research information found?

The large number of general and specialist journals produced around the world precludes the searching for individual articles by hand. Journal indexes have therefore been converted onto electronic databases to facilitate the process of finding research studies. Databases tend to gather together articles within the same specified subject categories, for example engineering, biology, sociology, history, medicine or agriculture. Most collect similar information about each included article. This is usually the title, author, where it was published (the journal, year, volume, issue and page numbers) and the short abstract/summary if available. They do not normally contain the full text of the whole article. These databases are known as 'bibliographic' databases.

Each individual journal article in a database is often referred to as a 'record' and each section of an article (title, author, abstract, etc.) is called a 'field'. Each new field starts with a two-letter code to make it clearly identifiable.

For example, a typical record in a bibliographic database, might look something like this:

TI: The joys of nursing
AU: Anybody G. C., Somebody H. L., Other A. N.
SO: Supernurse, 1997, 15 (2); 378–84
PY: 1997
AB: There have been many campaigns over recent years to boost the recruitment of young people into the nursing profession. These have taken a variety of approaches and focused on different aspects of the job, from how challenging nursing is – to the rewards of watching a patient recover from illness/injury. This paper looks at the positive images of nursing portrayed in these advertising campaigns and compares them with the reality as perceived by nurses currently employed.
UI: SN9725938

Databases are produced in a variety of formats: CD-ROM versions, world wide web/internet versions, or direct 'on-line' access options. Increasingly, in many organisations (such as hospitals) databases are 'networked' onto all the PCs of the institution. Databases are mainly produced by commercial companies so they are not usually free of charge. An organisation will have to pay for access to a database and this can limit the range made available for searching.

Getting help

Before attempting any literature searching, find out what help and support is available. Hospital libraries may provide direct training on searching databases, or more general guidance and support. Librarians advise on the databases and other resources available and may provide written instructions or have self-help tutorials.

Basic search principles

Although databases are produced by different companies and contain information on different subjects, they all tend to use the same approach when it comes to searching. This section looks at some basic theory that can be applied to searching different databases. The key principle in searching is to match words that describe a question/topic of interest with journal articles containing the same (or very similar) words. The idea is that these articles will be investigating/discussing the topic/question of interest.

Analysing the question

When starting a literature search, it is important to have a clear question in mind, so the exact information required can be identified. The first step in developing a search strategy is to break a question down into its key components (see the PICO question formulation process described in Chapter 2). It is necessary to think about the population, the treatments/interventions, any comparison interventions and specific outcomes covered by a question. Two examples are given in Box 3.1.

Box 3.1 Two questions broken down into key components

Question 1: What is the best way to alleviate fear associated with needles and injections?

Population:	People with fear of needles
Intervention(s):	Behavioural
	Relaxation
	Distraction
	Hypnotherapy
	Education

Box 3.1 (*contd.*)

Comparison:	One intervention compared with another
Outcome:	Fear/anxiety reduced

Question 2: Do oral antibiotics/treatments enhance healing, or are topical dressings sufficient for treatment of leg ulcers in sickle cell disease?

Population:	People with sickle-cell disease leg ulcers
Intervention(s):	Oral treatments
	Topical treatments
Comparison:	Oral treatments in conjunction with topical treatments, compared to topical treatments alone
Outcome:	Improvement in ulcer (heals, area is reduced)

Generating a word list

Having established the key components of a question, a word list needs to be generated for each component. All the different synonyms and phrases that could be used to describe a component need to be listed. Plural as well as singular words, abbreviations, American spellings, possible hyphenation and any regularly used non-English language terms should be included. With a bit of brainstorming, it is possible to produce quite comprehensive lists for each component (Box 3.2).

Be cautious when using abbreviations. Sometimes the same abbreviation can be used to represent different terminology. For

Box 3.2 Suggested word lists for questions 1 and 2

Question 1

Population:	fear of needles, fear of syringes, fear of injection(s), phobia of needles, phobia of syringes, phobia of injection(s), fear of hyperdermic(s), phobia of hyperdermic(s)
Interventions:	behavio(u)r(al), education, relaxation, coping skills, psychological, counselling, hypnotherapy, hypnosis, psychotherapy, distraction, divert attention
Comparison:	(same as interventions)
Outcomes:	alleviation of fear, alleviation of stress, stress relief, calm, relaxed

Question 2

Population:	sickle cell leg ulcer(s), sickle-cell leg ulcer(s), sickle cell an(a)emia leg ulcer(s), sickle-cell an(a)emia leg ulcer(s), sickle cell disease leg ulcer(s), sickle-cell disease leg ulcer(s)
Interventions:	ointment, dressing(s), cream(s), topical application, topically applied, oral antibiotic(s), oral drug(s), oral application
Comparison:	(same as intervention)
Outcomes:	ulcer reduction, ulcer reduced, area of ulcer reduced, ulcer heals, ulcer healed over, ulcer reduction

example, BNF is used for the 'British Nutrition Foundation' as well as the 'British National Formulary', so it may pick up articles on the wrong topic. Searching for the abbreviation AIDS can cause particular problems, because it will identify articles looking at hearing aids, mobility aids, etc. Abbreviations are very useful to include, but a bit of care and thought can help avoid any obvious pitfalls.

Linking word lists (Boolean logic: AND, OR, NOT)

Once separate word lists have been generated, it is necessary to link those lists to get the combination of components needed for a question.

Linking word lists in searching is done using two concepts: AND and OR. AND combines words/phrases together, so that both must appear within one article to be found by a search (Figure 3.1). For example, for question 1 a search for 'needles AND fear' will only find articles containing both the words needles and fear. For question 2, a search for 'sickle cell disease AND leg ulcers' will only find articles containing both the phrases sickle cell disease and leg ulcers.

OR enables selection of any one of a number of specified words/phrases in a list, so that if either one or another specified word/phrase appears in an article, it will be found in a search (Figure 3.2). For example, for the 'intervention' terms from question 1, a search for 'behavioural OR behavioral OR behaviour OR behavior OR education OR relaxation OR hypnotherapy OR hypnosis OR distraction OR diverting attention' will find articles containing at least one of the words/phrases in the list. For question 2, a search for

Figure 3.1 **The Boolean operator AND only identifies articles containing both specified components**

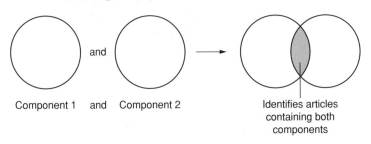

Component 1   and   Component 2   Identifies articles
                                          containing both
                                          components

Figure 3.2 **The Boolean operator OR identifies articles containing either specified component**

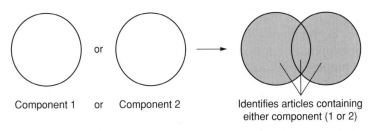

Component 1   or   Component 2   Identifies articles containing
                                          either component (1 or 2)

'ointment OR dressing OR dressings OR cream OR creams OR topical application OR topically applied' will find articles containing at least one of the words/phrases in the list. It is necessary to link all the individual terms/phrases in each word list, using OR, to avoid missing any articles that discuss that specific component.

It is also possible to exclude specific words/phrases from a search, so articles containing them will not be identified. This is done using the concept NOT (Figure 3.3). For example, for question 1 a search for 'fear of needles NOT fear of hospitals' will find articles containing the phrase 'fear of needles', which do not also contain the phrase 'fear of hospitals'. For question 2, a search for 'leg ulcer NOT pressure sore' will find articles containing the phrase 'leg ulcer', which do not also contain the phrase 'pressure sore'.

Be very cautious when using NOT, as it can inadvertently exclude articles that are relevant to a question.

AND, OR and NOT are also known as 'Boolean logic'. Searching by matching words and phrases in the general text of a record on a database is known as 'free text' searching.

Figure 3.3 The Boolean operator **NOT** identifies articles containing one specified component but not the other specified component

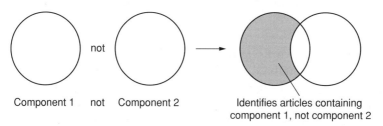

Component 1   not   Component 2   Identifies articles containing
                                          component 1, not component 2

Additional search tools commonly available

There are a few additional search tools that can help refine a basic search strategy as developed above.

Truncation

This is a shortcut device to save time, so all the different variations of a word do not have to be typed out as part of a search strategy. It works by finding the beginning of a word with any different ending on it. It is often denoted by a * or $ in databases. The 'help' option within the database will explain which symbol should be used. For example:

> child* would pick up child, children, childhood, etc.
> ulcer$ would pick up ulcer, ulcers, ulceration, ulcerated, etc.

Avoid using truncation after only a few letters at the start of a word – it can pick up more than expected. For example 'bab*' would pick up baby and babies, but also other words like baboon, babesiosis, babble, babesia, Babinski reflex, etc.

Wildcard

The 'wildcard' allows you to identify alternative spellings of the same word easily. The wildcard is inserted in the middle of a word where an extra letter, or alternative letter might be placed. When searched, spellings with any extra letter or different letter in that position will be identified. It is often denoted by a ? in databases. For example:

an?emia would pick up both anaemia and anemia
h?emoglobin would pick up both haemoglobin and hemoglobin
wom?n would pick up both woman and women

Index terms

These are keywords that are added onto each journal article included in a database, by the database producers. A specific topic is given just one keyword (also known as 'index term') to be used all the time. Index terms are usually quite specific so they accurately reflect the subject matter covered in an article. For example, every article that looks at breast cancer, breast carcinoma or breast tumours would be assigned one unique index term, which might be 'breast neoplasm'. It does not matter which specific words the authors of an article use to describe the topic, if the research investigates breast cancer, it will always be labelled with the index term 'breast neoplasm'. Each journal article will be assigned a number of appropriate index terms, to reflect the research it discusses.

This can aid searching, because instead of having to think of every way a component in a search could be described, the appropriate index term can be used instead. It also means that journal articles that mention a topic only in passing are not identified. Index terms are only given to describe subjects which form a large part of the investigation or discussion in the article.

A search that uses just index terms to find useful journal articles is known as a search on 'controlled vocabulary'.

A thesaurus

A thesaurus is a collection of all the index terms used by a database producer. It will usually be quite a complex listing, split into different subject areas with a hierarchical structure. A thesaurus can identify index terms of interest and in some databases the hierarchy structure can be used to search a range of index terms in one go.

Where to search first

Having clarified a question and identified the words necessary to search for relevant information, it is important to check whether anyone else has already gone through the research literature and published an answer to the question. For evidence-based health care questions, this means checking to see if anyone has done a 'systematic review' of the relevant research literature. (For more information on systematic reviews see Chapter 7.) The best place to check for systematic reviews in health care is on the 'Cochrane Library'.

The Cochrane Library

The Cochrane Library is not a standard bibliographic database and is, rather, a collection of separate databases (hence its title 'library').

Figure 3.4 **The opening screen of the Cochrane Library (from Update Software Ltd, with permission)**

List of the different databases on the Cochrane Library

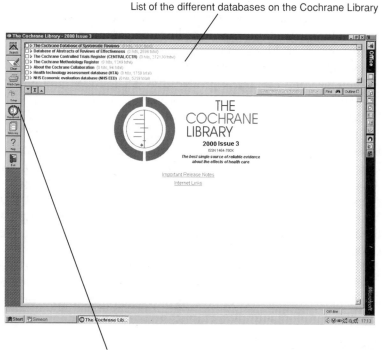

Tool bar of buttons, for searching, printing, to get help, etc.

The most useful databases for identifying systematic reviews are the Cochrane Database of Systematic Reviews (CDSR) and the Database of Abstracts of Reviews of Effectiveness (DARE). CDSR contains the full text of systematic reviews done through the auspices of the

Cochrane Collaboration. These reviews only include studies which are randomised controlled trials (RCTs) (the 'gold standard' for experimental research design). DARE contains abstracts of systematic reviews completed by groups outside of the Cochrane Collaboration, which use research information that will not always be randomised controlled trials. Each systematic review is described and then critically appraised. If no systematic reviews are found in CDSR, DARE should be checked. If nothing of interest is found there either, there is other information on the Cochrane Library that can be useful.

The Cochrane Controlled Trials Register (CCTR) and CENTRAL database is a bibliographic database of randomised controlled trials (and possibly randomised controlled trials) in health care. These trials have been identified by the Cochrane Collaboration. Looking in this database can help to identify good-quality research articles that are relevant to a question. The other databases on the Cochrane Library present information on health technology assessments, economic evaluations of health care interventions, systematic review methodology and the Cochrane Collaboration.

The Cochrane Library is produced as a CD-ROM and is also available on the internet. Most hospitals tend to have the CD-ROM version networked on their computer systems. An excellent self-training guide produced by the NHS Centre for Reviews and Dissemination (NHS CRD) is available and includes detailed instructions on how to search the Library and further details of the databases it contains. The guide is free to download from the website (http://www.york.ac.uk/inst/crd/cochlib.htm). The NHS CRD also has a designated Cochrane Library trainer, and many hospital libraries will also have their own guidelines and/or training on the Cochrane Library, as it is so relevant to the health care sector.

There are some other resources that try to do a similar job to the Cochrane Library (finding high-quality information only) that are available on the internet. See the section on 'Search systems on the internet' for more information (page 74).

Digests of evidence

Further resources that try to bring together the available good-quality evidence on a health care problem can be useful to check too. These include *Clinical Evidence*, which is produced as a book and on the internet (available on the National Electronic Library for Health to NHS Employees):

(http://www.clinicalevidence.) and *Health Evidence Bulletins Wales*, which are available on the internet (http://hebw.uwcm. ac.uk/).

Where to search next

If there are no systematic reviews or digests that already answer a question, or if some extra 'top-up' searching is required, the next place to look is in standard bibliographic databases that contain details of a wide range of journal articles.

In the health care/nursing field there are plenty of databases of interest. For example:

- MEDLINE (a general medical database, produced in the USA)
- CINAHL (Cumulative Index of Nursing and Allied Health Literature, a general nursing database, produced in the USA)
- Embase (a general medical database, produced in Europe – more foreign language material)
- BNI (British Nursing Index, a general nursing database).

See Appendix 3.1 (page 81) for further information.

All these databases are produced by different companies/organisations so they will often look different and contain different information, the specific searching tools available may vary and there will be variation between CD-ROM, internet and 'on-line' versions.

Which database you choose to search will depend on factors such as:

- The specific subject of a search
- Availability
- How easy/difficult it is to search.

It is helpful to find out as much as possible about any databases that are available (check search tools, etc.) and to do a quick test search to see how useful they are in practice.

Always make a note of which particular database(s) are searched, the years searched and the version(s) used, for each question or project that is undertaken.

An example search on the MEDLINE database

This next section looks at the process of undertaking a search on the MEDLINE database (the SilverPlatter CD-ROM version of the database). Question 1 from the Basic search principles section (Box 3.1) is used in building a search specifically designed for MEDLINE. Some controlled vocabulary searching (using index terms) as well as free text searching is used.

Step 1: checking what search tools are available

First check the search tools available in the database. This will usually be under the help information in the database (look for a 'help' button or heading), or in any library guidelines/instructions. Check which words the database uses for Boolean logic. They are often

Figure 3.5 **The opening search screen of MEDLINE on the SilverPlatter CD-ROM (from SilverPlatter Information Ltd and the US National Library of Medicine, with permission)**

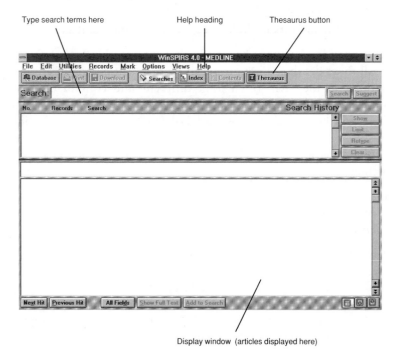

Type search terms here   Help heading   Thesaurus button

Display window (articles displayed here)

AND, OR and NOT, but not always. Check whether the terms are case sensitive. Also check for the symbol used for truncation and the wildcard, if these options are available and if a phrase has to be specified in any way, for example using quotation marks. For MEDLINE on SilverPlatter CD-ROM, the Boolean terms it uses are AND, OR and NOT; the truncation symbol is * and the wildcard symbol is ?. Phrases do not need to be specially identified in any way.

If the availability of an index and thesaurus has not already been established, again check the help information or any written instructions to clarify if these tools are offered. For MEDLINE on SilverPlatter CD-ROM, there is a thesaurus of indexing terms, known as MeSH™ (Medical Subject Headings) available for use. MeSH is a registered trademark of the United States National Library of Medicine.

Figure 3.6 **The thesaurus screen, after looking up the index term 'fear' (from SilverPlatter Information Ltd and the US National Library of Medicine, with permission)**

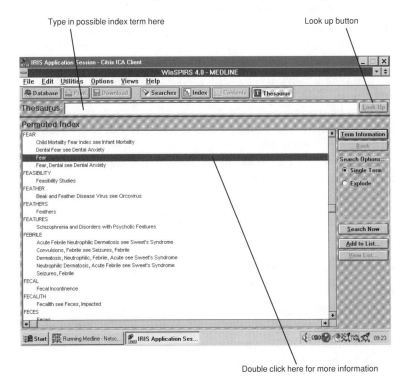

Type in possible index term here   Look up button

Double click here for more information

Step 2: using the index/thesaurus

To make use of any indexing terms in a search, it is necessary to identify those terms that correspond to the concepts identified in the original question. By clicking on the 'thesaurus button', a search can be done in the MEDLINE MeSH™ thesaurus to look for relevant terms (Figure 3.6). Type in the first concept and then click on the 'look up' button to get an alphabetical listing, which may have a heading or a close/exact match highlighted. (Click on a highlighted term to get a definition and see any more specific terms, if there are any.) If the highlighted term does not look relevant, scroll up or down the screen to see if there may be a useful index term. If nothing looks a reasonable match, look up a different description of the concept. If a useful match for a concept is found, make a note of it, so it can be used in the search. Sometimes there will not be a convenient index term or phrase available, so stop searching if nothing is identified after looking up a number of different descriptions.

Step 3: getting a search ready

Having checked through the details of the search tools and found some useful index terms to use, add that information into the written words/phrases list already prepared. It is a good idea to have a written plan to keep track of the search terms that will be typed in and the symbols that will be used. In this way, mistakes are less likely to be made.

The standard way of doing this is to write out the search as a series of steps, each step starting on a new line, with each new line being numbered. The final line of the search should bring together the combination of words you wish to find in the journal articles. This is also the standard format used for entering searches into a database (Boxes 3.3 and 3.4).

Box 3.3 Basic search plan for question 1 (written prior to checking index terms)

#1 fear OR phobia
#2 needles OR syringes OR injections OR injection OR hyperdermic OR hyperdermics
#3 #1 AND #2

Box 3.3 (*contd.*)

#4   hypnotherapy OR hypnosis OR psychotherapy OR
     behavioural OR behavioral
#5   behaviour OR behavior OR education OR coping skills OR
     counselling
#6   relaxation OR distraction OR divert attention
#7   #4 OR #5 OR #6
#8   #3 AND #7
#9   stress OR fear
#10 relief OR alleviation OR alleviated
#11 #9 AND #10
#12 calm OR relaxed
#13 #11 OR #12
#14 #8 AND #13

**Box 3.4 New enhanced search strategy for question 1,
specially written for MEDLINE SilverPlatter
CD-ROM**

#1   PHOBIC DISORDERS
#2   FEAR
#3   fear OR phobi*
#4   #1 OR #2 OR #3
#5   SYRINGES
#6   NEEDLES
#7   INJECTIONS
#8   needle* OR syringe* OR injection* OR hyperdermic*
#9   #5 OR #6 OR #7 OR #8
#10 HYPNOSIS OR PSYCHOTHERAPY
#11 RELAXATION TECHNIQUES OR BEHAVIOR THERAPY
#12 COUNSELING OR ADAPTATION, PSYCHOLOGICAL
#13 hypnosis OR hypnotherapy OR psychotherapy OR behavio?r
#14 behavio?ral OR counsell* OR coping skill* OR relax*
#15 distract* OR divert* attention
#16 #10 OR #11 OR #12 OR #13 OR #14 OR #15
#17 stress OR fear
#18 relief OR alleviat*
#19 #17 AND #18
#20 calm* OR relax*

Box 3.4   (*contd.*)
#21 #19 OR #20
#22 #4 AND #9
#23 #22 AND #16
#24 #21 AND #23

In Boxes 3.3 and 3.4 the controlled vocabulary (index terms and Boolean terms) has been written using capital letters and the free text terms of the search have been written in lower case. This makes them easier to differentiate.

Step 4: entering your search strategy onto the database

At this point the search strategy is ready to be entered.

Figure 3.7 **The search screen, after searching for some free text (from SilverPlatter Information Ltd and the US National Library of Medicine, with permission)**

Drops down from search box, when search finished

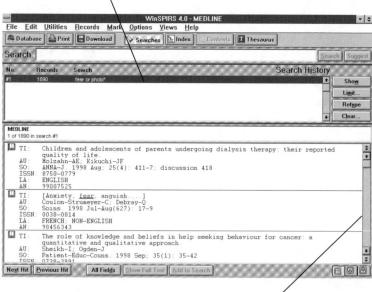

Scroll up and down to view records identified

Free text

To enter in free text, type in a line of the strategy in the blank search box (leaving out the line number at the beginning). Once it is typed in, click on the search button and the database will start looking for any journal articles containing the words (or combination of words) specified (Figure 3.7).

Index term

To enter an index term, go into the thesaurus (via the 'thesaurus' button) and search for the term to be used. Once the index term is found and is highlighted, click on the 'search now' button and a search will be made to find the articles assigned that term in the database. (Before the search process is started, a box asking about subheadings may appear. Just choose 'all subheadings' and the search process should continue.) The main search screen automatically returns to show the results of the search (Figure 3.8).

Figure 3.8 **The search screen, after searching for an index term (from SilverPlatter Information Ltd and the US National Library of Medicine, with permission)**

Index term just searched, appears here

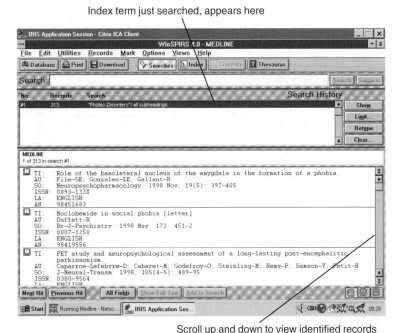

Scroll up and down to view identified records

Once the search has been completed, the free text or index term appears in the 'search history' box and is automatically given the appropriate line number (#1, #2, etc.). The number of journal articles matching that search line is displayed. This process is repeated with each new search line and in this way the search strategy written on paper is duplicated line by line in the 'search history' box on the screen (Figure 3.9).

When all the search strategy has been typed in, the final line should give the group of journal articles containing the information required. Depending on how many journal articles are in that final group, they can be assessed one by one on screen, but usually it is necessary to print them out, or save them onto a floppy disk. Look for a 'print' button or a 'save/download' button to do this. There is usually the choice of which records to print/save and

Figure 3.9 **The search screen, showing the 'search history' box replicating, line by line, the search strategy that has been searched so far (from SilverPlatter Information Ltd and the US National Library of Medicine, with permission)**

Search strategy reproduced here

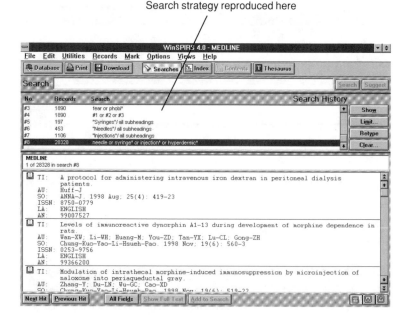

the specific fields to be included as well. Check the 'help information' for full details. The articles can then be viewed later at leisure. This completes the procedure for doing a basic search on MEDLINE SilverPlatter CD-ROM. Most databases follow this pattern of having to search specifically for index terms to be used in a search. However, CD-ROM and internet databases supplied by the company Ovid operate differently. When searching an Ovid version of MEDLINE, using the main search box, the search system automatically goes to the thesaurus and suggests an index term to use. This is known as 'mapping' – the text typed in is 'mapped' onto an index or thesaurus term. To search more generally for words occurring anywhere in an article, it is necessary to specify the 'free text/text word' option and search there (or turn off the mapping function, before searching).

Common queries regarding searching

In what order should search terms be typed/listed in a search strategy?

There are no strict rules on how a search should be typed in or written out. Things can be done in any order; words/phrases can be split up, so there are more lines in a search; or lumped together so there are fewer lines overall. As long as the logic of each step is correct and it arrives at the same final combination of words in the last line, the result should be the same.

Is it better to use free text or controlled vocabulary (index terms)?

Which should be used depends on the search to be done. Controlled vocabulary using index terms is more accurate, because there is less need to think about all the different terminology that could be used to describe an illness or population, etc. However, not all databases have indexing and it can take a while to find the index terms to use. (This is why Ovid versions of databases direct you to index terms as the default option – to try to make things easier for novice searchers.) Most people start searching using the free text approach, but where a database has controlled vocabulary, it is best to try and use it if possible. If a more thorough search is required, both types need to be used (as index terms can be assigned incorrectly).

So for simple searches: start with free text searching, experimenting with controlled vocabulary, then use controlled vocabulary as soon as it feels comfortable. For thorough searches use both types of search method to find as much as possible.

How do you know when all the relevant journal articles in a database have been found?

Unfortunately, there is no way to know if everything of interest has been found or not. Most bibliographic databases expand very quickly to contain thousands of articles, because there are so many journal papers being published and added to the databases all the time. No one can keep track of precisely the subjects being covered. The idea of searching is to maximise the relevant articles that are found, whilst at the same time minimising the irrelevant material.

Finding 'most' of the useful information in a database is the best that can be hoped for. Searching is a pragmatic exercise and there is always the possibility that something will have been missed unintentionally, regardless of the experience of the searcher.

Tips for more advanced users

There are a number of further tools and additional ways to prepare a strategy that will help to manage different search results.

Proximity operators

Some database systems have tools available that allow searching for a number of words in the same sentence, or paragraph, etc. Some systems allow you to specify exactly how close two words need to be (e.g. within six words of each other). These are called proximity operators.

For example a database may use WITH to find words/phrases contained in the same sentence and NEAR to find words/phrases contained in the same paragraph. The search 'midwife WITH care-team' would find articles containing at least one sentence with both midwife and care-team in it, and 'sickle cell NEAR leg ulcer' would find articles containing a paragraph with both sickle cell and leg ulcer in it.

These sorts of tools are most useful in databases where the majority of records have an abstract or summary.

Limiting to specific fields

Most database systems allow searches for information in the specific 'fields' of each journal article. This enables searches for words only in the title, articles by a specific author, or in a certain journal. Most systems tend to give each field in any article an abbreviated code, which can be used when searching. Check the 'help information' in a database to find out about the limiting options and how to select them.

For example, in databases where the codes TI, AU, SO and AB are used to identify the fields Title, Author, Source and Abstract, the search 'injections in TI' would find articles with the word injections in the title field, 'Bloggs.au' would find articles with the word Bloggs in the author field, and 'nurse in SO' would find articles with the word nurse in the source field.

Using the thesaurus

As well as helping to identify index terms of interest, a thesaurus can also allow searching of a group of related index terms in one go. For example, if you were interested in treatments for leg ulcers, you may find a number of indexing terms that are of interest listed in the thesaurus, for example, 'leg ulcers', 'leg pressure sores', 'diabetic foot ulcers', 'foot ulcers', etc. Each of these terms could be added separately into a search strategy, but it would save time if all the indexing terms related to leg ulcers could be added in one step. This is possible in many thesauri because index terms are listed in a hierarchy.

Basic structure of a thesaurus

A thesaurus orders index terms into hierarchical lists, with general terms (like dermatology, surgery, orthopaedics, community care, etc.) at the top and more precise, specific terms (on the same subject) underneath (like psoriasis, key hole surgery, fractured neck of femur, etc.). When written out, these lists are often called tree structures (the lists 'branch out' rather like a tree). For example, Box 3.5 shows what a section of a medical/health care thesaurus might look like. Terms at the top of a list are called 'broader terms' and those indented underneath are known as 'narrower' terms. In the example in Box 3.5, 'haemoglobinopathies' is a broader term

Box 3.5   Example showing what a section of a thesaurus might look like

Cardio-pulmonary system
　Blood
　　Blood disorders
　　　Parasitic infections
　　　Blood pressure disorders
　　　　Hypertension
　　　　Hypotension
　　　Blood cell disorders
　　　Coagulopathies
　　　　Haemophilia A
　　　　Haemophilia B
　　　　Von Willebrand's disease
　　　Haemoglobinopathies
　　　　Thalassaemia
　　　　Sickle cell anaemia
　　　　　Vaso-occlusive crisis
　　　　　Sickle cell leg ulcers

than 'thalassaemia' and 'sickle cell anaemia', whereas 'thalassaemia' and 'sickle cell anaemia' are narrower terms of 'haemoglobinopathies'. Following the same pattern, 'haemoglobinopathies' is a narrower term of 'blood disorders'.

Exploding index terms

To find all the information related to 'blood', for example, a search should be done on the index term blood and all the other blood-related conditions or issues in the index as well. This involves searching for blood and all its narrower terms in the thesaurus. To do this in one step is called 'exploding' an index term. By highlighting 'blood' in the thesaurus of the database and then selecting the 'explode button' (before pressing the search button) the search will automatically search blood and all the narrower terms indented underneath it (Figure 3.10).

For example, returning to the section of the thesaurus in the previous example, to search for anything on blood disorders, explod-

Figure 3.10 **The thesaurus screen from the MEDLINE SilverPlatter CD-ROM**, showing the tree structure for the index term 'fear'. If we 'explode' the term fear, we will search for articles assigned the index terms fear, dental anxiety and panic (from SilverPlatter Information Ltd. and the **US** National Library of Medicine, with permission)

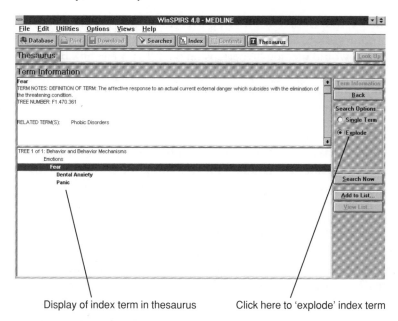

Display of index term in thesaurus   Click here to 'explode' index term

ing the index term 'blood disorders' would automatically search the following index terms:

Blood disorders
   Parasitic infections
   Blood pressure disorders
      Hypertension
      Hypotension
   Blood cell disorders
   Coagulopathies
      Haemophilia A
      Haemophilia B
      Von Willebrand's disease

Haemoglobinopathies
    Thalassaemia
    Sickle cell anaemia
        Vaso-occlusive crisis
        Sickle cell leg ulcers

The explode function picks up everything *beneath and indented to the right* of the exploded term. Exploding 'blood pressure disorders' would include 'hypertension' and 'hypotension', but would not pick up 'blood cell disorders', 'coagulopathies' or 'haemoglobinopathies'. This is because they are directly under 'blood pressure disorders' and not indented to the right.

Subheadings

To help make an index term even more precise, or tailored to a specific aspect, some systems include an option to search an index term with certain subheadings attached. Subheadings are generally categories such as diagnosis, prevention, adverse reactions, epidemiology, prognosis, surgery, etc. When an index term is assigned to an article, any appropriate subheadings will be linked to the term as well. If it is certain that the search only needs to focus on a narrow aspect of an index term, choosing the appropriate subheading(s) (rather than all of them) will limit the search to just the index term with that subheading attached. The MeSH™ thesaurus used on MEDLINE is an example of a database that has a subheading option.

Saving search strategies

Many database systems allow a completed search history to be saved, so the search can be run again, without having to type everything out all over again. Whilst this may not be a problem for short searches, once a search builds up a number of lines it can be very helpful to use this facility. Check the 'help information' on the database to find out how to go about saving a search strategy.

Too many or too few articles

If too many articles are found it may be necessary to narrow down a search to make it more accurate. Use more precise index terms or link them to specific subheadings; or perhaps search over a fewer number of years. It may be necessary to break up a broad subject into a series of questions, so the volume of information available can be better managed.

If only a few articles of interest are found, it may be necessary to widen out a search, so it is not so precise. Use broader index terms linked to all subheadings, or more general free text terms. If information is required on a very specific question, a low search result could mean little research has been done on that exact topic. It may be necessary to go back to the original question to see if it can be expanded.

When to stop searching

This very much depends on the objectives of a search. If a comprehensive literature review/survey is required, it needs to be very thorough, so a number of different databases should be searched to get as much useful material as possible. If a few conflicting articles are required on a topic to get an 'evidence base' debate going, or to stimulate discussion about treatment options, etc., a quick search on one database may be quite sufficient. If an up-to-date systematic review on a question has been identified, searching may be stopped after looking at the Cochrane Library.

The amount of searching done will also be influenced by the resources that are available: the time and databases available, the number of people involved in searching, etc. If comprehensive searches are done on a number of different databases, there will be gradually diminishing returns. The same journal articles will reappear each time and the volume of new articles identified will decrease. There will come a point when the effort involved in searching is not worth the tiny reward of new material found.

There is no right or wrong answer on when to stop searching. As with many aspects of the search process it is a pragmatic decision. The main thing is to be explicit about which databases have been searched. This avoids any confusion and allows a search to be accurately updated or expanded by looking in different databases.

Searching for a systematic review

Completing a systematic review is increasingly becoming part of higher degree courses and specialist training programmes.

Systematic reviews done in these settings will be restricted by time and the resources available. This is true for the searching component of the review, as well as the other parts. The searching required to complete a piece of coursework will be a lot less than that required to do a comprehensive systematic review in earnest. However, there are still a few issues to consider that may enhance a standard search.

Unpublished information

There is an increasing awareness that not all good-quality research work is published in professional journals. For various reasons, much interesting research is not reported in this way. In order to try to identify as many relevant studies as possible, there is often a requirement when undertaking a systematic review to go through conference proceedings, theses or project reports etc. to see if any additional information can be found. Also, many journals are not included in electronic databases. If there is a journal that covers research relevant to a review but that is not included in the databases being searched, it may necessitate going through issues of the journal by hand.

This sort of extra work cannot be done when time is restricted. However, the Cochrane Collaboration has a commitment to try and find unpublished RCTs, so its review groups search conference proceedings and go through journals by hand in an effort to do this. Any extra RCTs found in this way are published on the CCTR/CENTRAL database on the Cochrane Library. This means that searching this database on the Cochrane Library provides a quick and practical solution for finding unpublished information for a review.

Research in progress

Another aspect of searching in a systematic review is the need to identify any research that is in progress or about to be completed that could be relevant to the review. The main resource in this area for UK-based clinical research is the National Research Register (NRR) produced by the Department of Health (DoH). It aims to contain details of all the research being undertaken in the NHS, to help keep track of what is going on and to avoid any unnecessary duplication. Also from the DoH is the Research Findings

Electronic Register (ReFeR), which provides information on the results of DoH-funded research projects as they are just completed. There are also various lists appearing on the internet covering research in progress, such as the Current Controlled Trials site, which aims to identify RCTs that are underway. Having a quick look at these sorts of resources adds another aspect to a systematic review search.

The NRR can be found at:
http://www.update-software.com/National/nrr-frame.html
(It is also issued as a CD-ROM, so may be available in hospital libraries or networked onto hospital PCs).

ReFeR can be found at:
http://www.doh.gov.uk/research/rd3/information/findings.htm

Current Controlled Trials can be found at:
http://controlled-trials.com

Searching for an extensive systematic review

Undertaking the searching for a fully fledged systematic review (with funding, longer time-scale, etc.) is not something that should be done lightly. It does require a lot of searching experience and knowledge of available resources. Budgeting is necessary to ensure all searching-related activities can be completed (obtaining and translating articles, as well as accessing databases) and the time-scale must allow for searching any conferences or journal titles by hand.

More information on this type of extensive searching can be found in:

NHS CRD Report 4. Undertaking Systematic Reviews of Research on Effectiveness – CRD Guidance for Carrying out or Commissioning Reviews, 2nd edn. Phase 3: Identification of Research; Appendix I: Literature Searching. http://www.york.ac.uk/inst/crd/report4.htm

'Cochrane Reviewer's Handbook' (5: Locating and Selecting Studies) available on the Cochrane Library CD-ROM.

NHS CRD Information Service. Finding Studies for Systematic Reviews: a Basic Checklist for Researchers. http://www.york.ac.uk/ inst/crd/infoserv.htm (under Information Resources).

Box 3.6 Key points to remember about searching electronic databases

1. Get help
   Attend training sessions in hospital/university libraries. Find out about support for searching in general.
2. Prepare the search
   Sort out the question/topic, generate word lists, have a draft search planned.
3. Find out more
   What database(s) might be useful to search, what tools they have (truncation, thesaurus, etc.), how those tools are used – check the 'help' information and any written guidelines.
4. Decide which database to search
   Do a brief test search, check ease of searching, make sure all useful information is available.
5. Prepare the final search strategy
   Add in index terms, truncation symbols, etc. for the database to be searched.
6. Do the search
   Select index terms, type in free text terms. Get the final set of useful records at the end.
7. Print or save the final set of articles
   Print/save the records to look at later on.
8. Keep a record of the resources searched
   Make a note of the database, the version used (Ovid CD-ROM, SilverPlatter on the internet, etc.), the years searched and the date the search was done.
9. Keep a record of the search strategy
   Make sure a copy is kept, so the exact details are available for future reference.
10. If searching for systematic review, access sources of unpublished and on-going research.

The internet

The internet is often referred to as the 'world wide web', and it is useful to think of it in this way to illustrate its positive and negative aspects. Like a spider on its web, the internet can provide an invisible link between isolated points, enabling seamless travel to relevant sources without having to follow laborious routes, allowing movement from resource to resource and back again easily and quickly. However, the internet can also appear to be an unrelated tangle of too much information – just as a web is a trap for an unwary fly. There are so many sites of possible interest it is easy to get completely lost and overwhelmed. The internet can be a very confusing and frustrating tool to use, as well as an extremely useful collection of information resources.

The other issue of concern is the lack of quality control. The internet is not owned or governed by any one company or organisation. Any individual with the appropriate expertise and equipment can create a 'web page' and make it available on the internet. There is no registration required, no standards that have to be met and nobody has to be informed. Web pages appear and disappear all the time. People can choose to provide accurate, useful and honest web pages, or not. Hence the concern over offensive, illegal and deliberately misleading information that can appear on the world wide web. The internet is a vast international collection of information and misinformation that people choose to make available.

Searching the internet

To undertake an organised search for journal articles, use the same sort of bibliographic databases as those discussed in the rest of the chapter. This means using the internet versions of databases (some of which need to be paid for). MEDLINE is the main database that is available free of charge on the internet. PubMed is the version which comes direct from the creators of MEDLINE (the National Library of Medicine in the USA), but there are a number of other versions that are available. Hospital/university libraries should be able to advise about any bibliographic databases they subscribe to on the internet.

Search systems on the internet

In the area of evidence-based health care information, there are some useful search systems which search websites that list articles and other publications related to evidence-based health care.

TRIP (Turning Research into Practice) database

TRIP searches a broad range of evidence-based health care-related websites including Effective Healthcare Bulletins, NHS CRD Reports, Bandolier, the Cochrane Library databases and many others. The search screen is very simple to use. Just type in the word or phrase to be identified, when the search has been completed a list of relevant items is presented, with the name of the resource in which they were found. Click on items one by one to view them. The TRIP database can be searched at: http://www.tripdatabase.com/

SUMSearch

This is a search system devised by the University of Texas, Health Science Center at San Antonio. When search term(s) are typed in, this system will automatically check (internet versions of) MEDLINE, DARE, the National Guideline Clearinghouse from the Agency for Health Care Policy and Research (AHCPR), an on-line textbook (usually the Merck Manual) and a few other databases depending on the topic. It uses the MeSH™ (MEDLINE) thesaurus, so index terms can be used to search as well as free text. The search screen is straightforward to use and the system makes suggestions to help produce an accurate search. Search results are split into two types: broad/general discussions of the topic, or systematic reviews and original research. SUMSearch can be found at: http://sumsearch.uthscsa.edu/cgi-bin/SUMSearch.exe

Searching the internet more generally

To search the internet more generally for sites with any information related to a specific disease/illness or intervention, there are a number of different 'search engines' and 'meta-search engines' that can be used. They tend to use a simple approach, searching for any word or phrase that is specified. Typical search engines include: Google, Alta Vista, Yahoo, Lycos, etc. and typical meta-search engines include: SavvySearch, MetaCrawler, etc.

These systems trawl through web pages trying to find useful resources. Unfortunately, the result is often a list of thousands of sites to go through. Whilst this can be an interesting way to investigate what is on the internet, it is not the most efficient way to find useful information, especially if you are new to the internet or have limited time available. It is much easier to start off by using sites that give directions to quality-assessed and/or useful information. These usually take the form of recommended lists of 'gateway' sites, which are regularly updated and expanded as required.

Gateway sites

The most obvious sort of 'gateway' point is that provided on the web page of an organisation. Many university and hospital sites (often listed on the library/information service pages) include links to key websites considered reliable and useful to staff and students.

There are also some subject-specific 'gateway' sites, set up to serve groups of academics, researchers, students and others wanting information in that field. These are usually funded through academic research grants or projects and are available for anyone to use (with no charge). A number of these gateways are relevant to the health care sector.

OMNI (Organising Medical Networked Information)

This gateway is designed to direct viewers to health and medicine web pages, that have been assessed and met the desired quality standard. It has a section dedicated to MEDLINE sites on the web, giving an outline of what each site provides and often a review of the site from someone who has recently used it. It also provides some self-help tutorials on searching the internet, as well as links to sites that match its quality criteria. OMNI can be found at: http://omni.ac.uk/

NMAP (Nursing, Midwifery and Allied health Professions)

This gateway is a recent development that focuses specifically on identifying quality websites related to nursing, midwifery and the allied health professions. NMAP can be found at: http://nmap. ac.uk/

Both OMNI and NMAP form part of the BIOME group of gateways, which cover a range of topics in the biological sciences.

SOSIG (Social Science Information Gateway)

This is not part of the BIOME group, but aims to provide an equivalent resource for those interested in the social sciences. Of particular relevance to health care is the coverage of psychology (including mental health), social welfare (including community care and carers) and education. SOSIG can be found at: http://www.sosig.ac.uk/

Lists

Some groups provide lists of websites on certain subject areas to help people identify sites of possible interest. For evidence-based health care, there is an excellent list provided by ScHARR (the School of Health and Related Research), at Sheffield University, known as 'Netting the Evidence – A ScHARR Introduction to Evidence Based Practice on the Internet'. It consists of a list of evidence-based health care websites, each with an accompanying description, providing very useful background about each site. 'Netting the Evidence' can be found at: http://www.shef.ac.uk/ ~scharr/ir/netting.html

Links

The other approach to finding sites of interest is to go to the sites of organisations you already know about. Most professional bodies, research groups and charities have web pages, usually with a list of links to other websites that they think will be useful and of interest to their members and readers of their web page.

In evidence-based health care there are a number of organisations, such as the NHS Centre for Reviews and Dissemination, the Cochrane Collaboration, the Centre for Evidence Based

Nursing, etc., which have web pages. In the nursing field there are sites for the Royal College of Nursing, the Royal College of Midwives, etc. By visiting these organisation web pages, further suggestions of other places to look for relevant information may be found.

Last, but by no means least, is the National electronic Library for Health (NeLH), a comprehensive website providing a wealth of information, and access to most of the resources listed above. The NeLH can be found at: http://www.nelh.nhs.uk

See Appendix 3.2 (page 84) for further information.

Books and journals

There are a variety of publications discussing internet resources on health care and providing guidance for users. Whilst printed resources can become out of date quite quickly (especially when considering an ever changing environment like the internet), they are another means to get ideas or advice on websites that might be worth investigating.

For example:

Pallen Mark 1998 Guide to the internet: an introduction for healthcare professionals, 2nd edn. London: BMJ Publishing

Anon 1999 Health Net: a health and wellness guide to the internet, 2nd edn. London: McGraw-Hill

Kiley Robert 1999 Medical information on the internet: a guide for health professionals, 2nd edn. Edinburgh: Churchill Livingstone

Nicoll Leslie H 1998 Computers in nursing's nurses' guide to the internet, 2nd edn. Philadelphia: Lippincott

A few specialist newsletters/journals are also starting to appear, looking at the internet for health care professionals. These provide a way to keep track of new websites and developments. Two such publications are *Health on the Internet* and *Internet Medicine*.

Hospital and university libraries are the first place to look for any relevant books and/or journal titles about the internet.

Further information on using the internet

Training and teaching tools available on the internet to help novice users find out more about searching and using internet resources in general include:

Bare Bones, from the University of South Carolina, Beaufort Library. This provides a basic tutorial on searching the internet. It can be found at: http://www.sc.edu/beaufort/library/bones. html

Internet Medic (available from the OMNI site). This is a teach-yourself tutorial on information skills for the internet. It can be found at: http://omni.ac.uk/vts/medic/

There are also a large number of general publications available on how to use the internet (*Idiot's Guides* etc.). Hospital and university libraries may have a few books like this available to borrow.

Box 3.7 Key points to remember about searching the internet

1. The internet is a collection of all sorts of information. It has no quality control and no rules or regulations, so as well as extremely useful information, there may also be misleading or incorrect information.
2. To search for journal articles, use internet versions of established bibliographic databases (organisations may have to pay for access).
3. For evidence-based health care information (articles, reports and other documentation) on the internet, try the search systems TRIP or SUMSearch.
4. For directions to quality-assessed websites, or suggestions of particularly useful websites, use 'gateway' sites or subject lists or links compiled by reliable groups/ organisations.
5. For other ideas of useful internet resources, check libraries for any publications covering health care sites on the internet (books or newsletters/journals).

Box 3.7 (*contd.*)

6. To do some very broad searching, probably identifying thousands of websites of variable quality, use general internet search engines or meta-search engines.

Further reading

These are general articles about searching the health care literature aimed at the beginner/intermediate. As far as possible, they are recent and directed at a nursing audience. They should give more advice and ideas on how to approach literature searching in the clinical setting.

Cooke A 1999 Quality of health and medical information on the internet. British Journal of Clinical Governance 4(4): 155–160

Cullum N 2000 Users' guides to the nursing literature: an introduction. Evidence-Based Nursing 3: 71–72

Glanville J, Haines M, Auston I 1998 Finding information on clinical effectiveness. British Medical Journal 317: 200–203

Hendry C, Farley A 1998 Reviewing the literature: a guide for students. Nursing Standard 12(44): 46–48

Hunt DL, Haynes RB, Browman GP 1998 Searching the medical literature for the best evidence to solve clinical questions. Annals of Oncology 9(4): 377–383

Hunt DL, Jaeschhke R, McKibbon KA 2000 Users' guides to the medical literature: XXI using electronic health information resources in evidence-based practice. Journal of the American Medical Association 283(14): 1875–1879

Lowe HJ, Barnett GO 1994 Understanding and using the Medical Subject Headings (MeSH) vocabulary to perform literature searches. Journal of the American Medical Association 271(14): 1103–1108

NHS Centre for Reviews and Dissemination 2001 Accessing the evidence on clinical effectiveness. Effectiveness Matters 5(1). Available at: http://www.york.ac.uk/inst/crd/em51.htm

McKibbon KA, Marks S 1998 Searching for the best evidence: part 1: where to look. Evidence-Based Nursing 1(3): 68–69

McKibbon KA, Marks S 1998 Searching for the best evidence: part 2: searching CINAHL and Medline. Evidence-Based Nursing 1(4): 105–107

Sindhu F, Dickson R 1997 The complexity of searching the literature. International Journal of Nursing Practice 3(4): 211–217

Sindhu F, Dickson R 1997 Literature searching for systematic reviews. Nursing Standard 11(41): 40–42

Thompson C 1999 Searching for the evidence. Nursing Times/ Learning Curve 3(3): 12–13

Appendix 3.1
Electronic databases

This is by no means a comprehensive list, but a selection that is most likely to be available on hospital or university computer networks.

General medical

MEDLINE
: Produced by the National Library of Medicine (NLM) in the USA. Contains information from 1966 onwards. Uses index terms and has a thesaurus (MeSH™). It has a USA and English language bias. Very widely available.

Embase
: Produced by Elsevier Science, based in the Netherlands. Contains information from 1974 onwards. Uses index terms and a thesaurus (known as Emtree). Has a European bias and more emphasis on pharmaceutical information.

Nursing

CINAHL
: Cumulative Index to Nursing and Allied Literature, produced in the USA. Contains information from 1982 onwards. Uses index terms and has a thesaurus (called the Subject Heading List). See website: http://www.cinahl.com

BNI
: British Nursing Index, produced in the UK. Contains information from 1994 onwards. Consolidates from 1994, the British Midwifery Index and Nursing Bibliography and RCN Nurse ROM. Has a UK and English language bias.

Specialist

AIDSLINE
: Database of information on HIV and AIDS, produced by the NLM. Contains information from 1980 onwards.

CANCERLIT
: Database of information on cancer, produced by the US National Cancer Institute.

CABHealth	Database of information relating to human nutrition; parasitic, communicable (including AIDS/HIV) and tropical diseases; medicinal plants and public health. Contains information from 1973 onwards. Strong international and developing country coverage. Uses index terms and has a thesaurus (CAB thesaurus).
AMED	Allied and Complementary Medicine, produced by the British Library. Contains information from 1985 onwards. Includes physiotherapy, occupational therapy, rehabilitation and palliative care. Uses index terms and a thesaurus (AMED thesaurus, based on MeSH™).
PsycINFO	Produced by the American Psychological Association. Contains information from 1887 onwards. Covers all aspects of psychology. Uses index terms and a thesaurus (Thesaurus of Psychological Index Terms) for items dating from 1967 onwards.
LLBA	Linguistics and Language Behavior Abstracts. Contains information from 1981 onwards. Coverage includes speech, language and hearing pathology.

Health management

HealthSTAR	Produced by the NLM and American Hospitals Association (between 1978 and 1999). Contains information from 1975 onwards. Covers health care planning, policy and administration. Includes effectiveness of procedures, products and services and evaluation of patient outcomes.
HMIC	Health Management Information Consortium database. Produced in the UK, an amalgamation of databases from the Nuffield Institute of Health (University of Leeds), the Department of Health and the King's Fund.

Others

EBM Reviews	Database comprising of CDSR, DARE and the *American College of Physicians (ACP) Journal Club* journal.
Science Citation Index	Essentially an electronic version of the *Current Contents* publications covering scientific journals. Aims to add newly published articles on to the database promptly.
Social Science Citation Index	Sister publication to Science Citation Index, covering social science journals.

Appendix 3.2
Useful websites

National Electronic Library for Health

A first port of call for nurses employed by the NHS or by academic institutions within the UK is the NeLH http://www.nelh.nhs.uk. This site provides access to many of the organisations listed below.

Nursing organisations

For quality-assessed resources go to NMAP
http://nmap.ac.uk/

Royal College of Nursing
http://www.rcn.org.uk/

Royal College of Midwives
http://www.rcm.org.uk/

English National Board (ENB) for Nursing, Midwifery and Health Visiting
http://www.enb.org.uk/

National Board for Nursing, Midwifery and Health Visiting for Scotland (NBS)
http://www.nbs.org.uk/

Welsh National Board for Nursing, Midwifery and Health Visiting
http://www.wnb.org.uk/

National Board for Nursing, Midwifery and Health Visiting for Northern Ireland
http://www.n-i.nhs.uk/NBNI/index.htm

Midwives Information and Resource Service (MIDIRS) – a 'not for profit' organisation
http://www.midirs.org/

UK Central Council for Nursing, Midwifery and Health Visiting
http://www.ukcc.org.uk

Evidence-based practice organisations

For a comprehensive list, go to 'Netting the Evidence – A ScHARR Introduction to Evidence Based Practice on the Internet' http://www.shef.ac.uk/~scharr/ir/netting.html

Centre for Evidence Based Nursing
http://www.york.ac.uk/healthsciences

The Joanna Briggs Institute for Evidence based Nursing and Midwifery (Australia)
http://www.joannabriggs.edu.au

NHS Centre for Reviews and Dissemination (includes the publications *Effective Health Bulletins* and *Effectiveness Matters*)
http://www.york.ac.uk/inst/crd/

Cochrane Collaboration
http://www.cochrane.org

The Cochrane Library
http://www.update-software.com/cochrane/cochrane-frame.html

The Cochrane Library Self-training Guide and Notes
http://www.york.ac.uk/inst/crd/cochlib.htm

Clinical Evidence
http://www.clinicalevidence.com

Health Evidence Bulletins Wales
http://hebw.uwcm.ac.uk/

National Institute for Clinical Excellence (NICE)
http://www.nice.org.uk/nice-web/

The National Co-ordinating Centre for Health Technology Assessment
http://www.hta.nhsweb.nhs.uk

4

Critical appraisal 1: is the quality of the study good enough for you to use the findings?

Mark Newman and Tony Roberts

Key points

- Why is critical appraisal necessary?
- The principles of critical appraisal
- Identifying the appropriate research design for your clinical practice question
- Assessing the quality of studies answering questions about the effectiveness of therapy or interventions
- Assessing the quality of a study that asks a question about whether a particular diagnostic test or method of assessment works
- Assessing the quality of a study that asks questions about finding out the likely pattern and/or outcome of a particular health problem/disease
- Critical appraisal in practice.

This chapter should be read in conjunction with Chapter 5 (Critical appraisal 2: can the evidence be applied in your context?)

Introduction

Not all published research evidence can be used for making decisions about patient care. Deficiencies in research design can make an intervention look better than it really is (Cook & Campbell 1979). In addition, the location and subjects of a particular research study may affect the results in a unique way. It is therefore necessary to assess the quality, importance and applicability of any research evidence that is being consulted to answer a specific clinical question. The process used to do this is known as critical appraisal. Critical appraisal in this context is about answering a specific question related to the care of a specific patient or group of patients. The term critical appraisal is frequently used in relation to the conduct of a literature review for academic or educational purposes. Whilst the principles of critical appraisal are similar in both cases the difference in purpose is important. Educational or academic reviews are usually about gaining an understanding of the principles, issues and debates about a particular subject. The purpose of the critical appraisal for evidence-based practice is to decide whether the quality of a research study is good enough for the results it provides to be used to answer a question posed by a health care practitioner or patient.

Critical appraisal can be broken down into three distinct but related parts as illustrated in Figure 4.1. Over the past 20 years or so researchers and clinicians around the world have been working together to develop standard approaches to critical appraisal for evidence-based practice. This has led to the development of quality criteria to assess the design of research studies. These have been incor-

Figure 4.1 **The three aspects of critical appraisal for evidence-based practice**

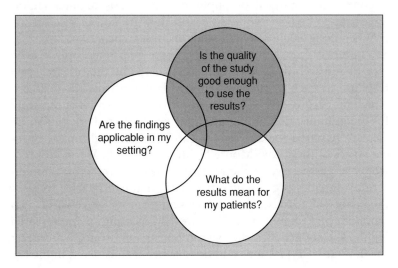

porated into critical appraisal checklists that make the process of assessing the quality of a study much easier.

This and the next chapter (Chapter 5) provide a set of tools that can be used for critical appraisal. The chapters also provide help in developing the skills and knowledge necessary to use these tools. The remainder of this chapter will consider how to assess whether the quality of the study is good enough for the results to be used (i.e. in shading in Figure 4.1). Chapter 5 addresses the other two aspects. Both chapters use practical examples to illustrate the process: clinical scenarios are used to generate clinical questions, then relevant published research papers are appraised. The same examples are used in both chapters. You will obtain more benefit from the examples if you obtain copies of the published research papers.

Is the quality of the study good enough for me to use the results?

The type of research evidence considered within these two chapters is that which is designed to find the answer to a specific question. One of the challenges that all researchers face in the design and conduct of research in real world settings is that of minimising bias. Bias refers to anything that erroneously distorts the conclusions of a study. In other words, any factor (for example the way the study is conducted, analysed or published) that leads to interventions appearing to be effective when in fact they are not, or vice versa.

When designing a research study the researchers have to consider a number of questions (Box 4.1). These questions apply in every type of research design. The decisions made by the researchers in response to each of these questions directly affects the degree to which the results of a study may be affected by bias. The strategies for the minimisation of bias are now well known. Different strategies are required for different research designs and for the different stages of the study (Moore & McQuay 2000). When looked at from the perspective of the research consumer these bias minimisation strategies become quality criteria that can be used to assess the quality of a study. The strategies adopted by the researchers to minimise bias should be evident in the reporting of the research. Figure 4.2 summarises the bias minimisation strategies (criteria) for the research questions and designs being considered in the two

> **Box 4.1 Questions to be considered in the design of a research study (after Blaikie 2000)**
>
> ■ What is the research question?
> ■ Which research design is the most appropriate to answer this question?
> ■ What is the appropriate sample and how will this be selected?
> ■ What will be measured?
> ■ How will the effects of the researcher be controlled?
> ■ How will the data be collected?
> ■ How will the data be analysed?

critical appraisal chapters. The criteria are explained in more detail in the worked examples later in the chapter.

Is the study design appropriate to the question?

As shown in Chapter 2, the process of critical appraisal for evidence-based practice starts with the formulation of a question that arises from clinical practice. For critical appraisal purposes clinical practice questions can, broadly speaking, be categorised into four types. In this and the following chapter, we are concerned with the three types of question referred to in Table 4.1 (see Chapter 6 for discussion of critical appraisal of questions requiring qualitative research designs).

For each type of question there is a corresponding 'most appropriate' research design (overall plan or structure used by the researcher) that can be used to answer the question with a known degree of precision and minimal risk of bias (Blaikie 2000). In this chapter we have focused on the optimal study design for three different types of questions, however, it is important to remember that there may be good reasons why researchers choose to use study designs that at first glance appear to be less appropriate for the research questions. Each research project presents unique challenges and a certain degree of flexibility is required by the researcher.

For each research design, specific criteria need to be considered. These criteria, listed in Figure 4.2, will be explored in more detail later on in the chapter.

Figure 4.2 **Criteria and questions for use in assessing the quality of research studies**

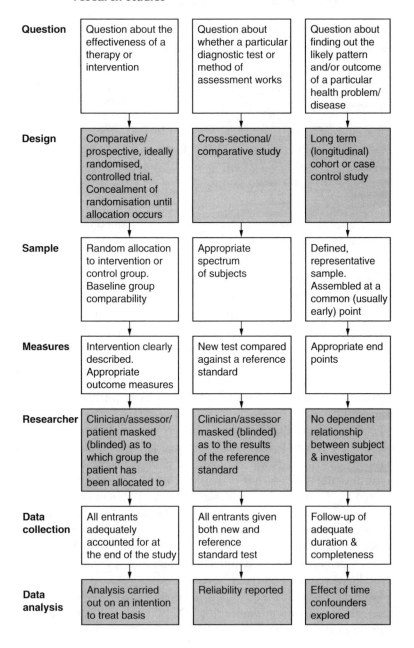

Question	Question about the effectiveness of a therapy or intervention	Question about whether a particular diagnostic test or method of assessment works	Question about finding out the likely pattern and/or outcome of a particular health problem/disease
Design	Comparative/ prospective, ideally randomised, controlled trial. Concealment of randomisation until allocation occurs	Cross-sectional/ comparative study	Long term (longitudinal) cohort or case control study
Sample	Random allocation to intervention or control group. Baseline group comparability	Appropriate spectrum of subjects	Defined, representative sample. Assembled at a common (usually early) point
Measures	Intervention clearly described. Appropriate outcome measures	New test compared against a reference standard	Appropriate end points
Researcher	Clinician/assessor/ patient masked (blinded) as to which group the patient has been allocated to	Clinician/assessor masked (blinded) as to the results of the reference standard	No dependent relationship between subject & investigator
Data collection	All entrants adequately accounted for at the end of the study	All entrants given both new and reference standard test	Follow-up of adequate duration & completeness
Data analysis	Analysis carried out on an intention to treat basis	Reliability reported	Effect of time confounders explored

Table 4.1 **Matching study design to questions**

Type of question	Example question	Research design
The effectiveness of a therapy or intervention	Does a nurse-led discharge package for children admitted with acute asthma reduce readmission rates?	Comparative/prospective randomised controlled trial
Finding out the likely pattern and/ or outcome of a particular health problem or disease (i.e. prognosis)	Are women oral contraceptive users who smoke at greater risk of myocardial infarction (MI)?	Cohort study: participants exposed to an agent (contraceptive pill) are followed forward in time to see if they develop an outcome (MI)
		Case-control study: participants with the condition (MI) are matched with controls (no MI), study looks back in time to identify exposure to an agent (contraceptive pill)
Whether a particular diagnostic test or method of assessment works	In primary care, does asking patients about feeling depressed and loss of interest accurately identify those who are clinically depressed?	Cross-sectional study where the 'new' test (or method of assessment) is compared with a reference standard test

In the case of questions about whether a particular diagnostic test or method of assessment works, a study design that compares the accuracy of the new test when used on people with and without the target condition against a reference standard will be most appropriate (Mant 1999a). Where the question is about the most likely outcome of a particular health problem (i.e. the prognosis), the most appropriate design will be one that measures relevant outcomes in individuals with (and perhaps without) the relevant condition over a sufficient period of time (Mant 1999b).

If the clinical question is about whether a particular intervention (e.g. a nurse-led discharge package) produces a certain outcome (e.g. decreased hospital stay), a study that compares length of hospital stay in a group receiving the intervention with length of hospital stay in a group not receiving the intervention is required.

There are a number of possible research designs that could be used for such a study, however large, multicentred randomised controlled trials (RCTs) are likely to give the best evidence of effectiveness (McKee et al 1998), provided they are conducted rigorously. Regardless of the type of study, a rigorous approach to the design, conduct, analysis and reporting stages of the study is important in view of the effect that each of these stages can have on the results. For example, randomised controlled trials with methodological shortfalls, such as failure to conceal from the patient and assessor the group to which the patient has been allocated, tend to overestimate treatment effects (Shultz et al 1995).

Systematic reviews

There has been an explosion in the amount of published research evidence, much of which is not easily accessible to practitioners. When searching for evidence, it is unlikely that all the studies that have been carried out with the aim of addressing a particular question will be identified. In addition, wading through large numbers of articles can be extremely time consuming and may not be an option for a busy practitioner. Where relevant studies are identified, their conclusions may differ, and this poses a dilemma for the person who is trying to find a solution to a problem. These are just some of the reasons for the growing interest in systematic reviews as a form of evidence. The systematic review differs from the traditional narrative review in that systematic, explicit methods are used to identify, assess and synthesise the information obtained. These 'secondary' research studies can help to overcome many of the practical and methodological limitations of individual studies (Mulrow 1994). To date, the majority of systematic reviews have focused on effectiveness of different interventions, where the study design used by the primary authors was the controlled trial, however systematic reviews of other types of study designs are also being conducted. In this chapter we have not looked at critical appraisal of systematic reviews, however critical appraisal checklists specific to systematic reviews are available. Chapter 7 provides more information.

The hierarchy of evidence

When looking for evidence about the effectiveness of interventions, properly conducted systematic reviews of RCTs or properly conducted RCTs provide the most powerful form of evidence. The process of randomisation means that the observed differences between the intervention group and the comparison group are more likely to be due to the intervention and not to other factors such as patient, nurse or doctor preference. There will, however, always be circumstances where randomisation may be inappropriate or impossible (Black 1990). An obvious example is studies about harm or prognosis. It would not be ethical to give subjects a substance that was thought to be hazardous to their health. In circumstances where there are genuine reasons for not randomising, studies with other designs have a vital role in providing evidence (McPherson 1994).

Evidence that some research designs are more powerful than others has given rise to the notion of a hierarchy of evidence (Peto 1993). Figure 4.3 illustrates this hierarchy for studies relating to effectiveness of therapies or interventions. The pyramid shape is used to illustrate the increasing risk of bias inherent in each research design. The hierarchy of evidence has sometimes been interpreted as suggesting that only questions about effectiveness are important and/or that randomised controlled trials are the only source of evidence (Castledine 1997, Maggs 1997). In reality, the hierarchy of evidence applies only to questions about the effectiveness of therapies or interventions and these are only one, albeit important, type of clinical question.

Figure 4.3 The hierarchy of evidence for questions about the effectiveness of an intervention/therapy

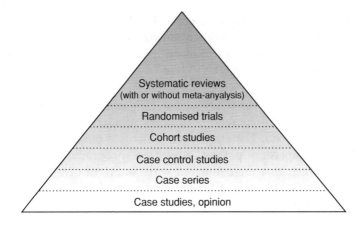

Systematic reviews
(with or without meta-anyalysis)

Randomised trials

Cohort studies

Case control studies

Case series

Case studies, opinion

Worked example 4.1: Assessing the quality of studies answering questions about the effectiveness of therapy or interventions

Scenario

You are part of the nursing team that works on a busy children's ward where one of the commonest reasons for admitting a child is acute asthma. At yesterday's case conference Sally Gibson, an 11 year old who has been admitted with acute asthma four times in the last 6 months, was discussed. The team discussed the different possible reasons for Sally's repeated admissions and there was some speculation that both Sally and her family may not be managing her medication and attacks of breathlessness very well. The team decides to find out more about whether educational interventions can be effective at reducing repeat admissions. One of the paediatricians recalls reading something about nurse-led discharge packages to help children and their family self-manage their asthma and promises to find the paper.

Your clinical practice question

Does a structured nurse-led discharge package result in reduced levels of readmission to hospital of children with acute asthma?

Finding the evidence

Your colleague supplies the following paper that looks as though it might be relevant:

> Wesseldine LJ, McCarthy P, Silverman M 1999 Structured discharge procedure for children admitted to hospital with acute asthma: a randomised controlled trial of nursing practice. Archives of Disease in Childhood 80: 110–114

The paper reports the results of a randomised controlled trial involving 160 children aged 2–16 years admitted for asthma over a 12-month period. The effects of a structured nurse-led discharge package comprising patient education programme and self-management plan were compared with 'standard care'. Outcome measures included rates of readmission to the accident and emergency department.

What is the quality of the study

Table 4.2 shows a worked example of the critical appraisal for the paper referenced above that applies the quality criteria for comparative study designs given in Figure 4.2. The quality criteria have been adapted from the critical appraisal guideline published in the Journal of the American Medical Association (referred to here as JAMA guides). Readers are directed to the JAMA guidelines for a more detailed discussion (Guyatt et al 1993).

Factors to consider when assessing the quality of a study

- The importance of randomisation has already been discussed: the aim is to ensure that, as far as possible, the two groups are similar apart from the intervention. This means that any difference in outcome between the two groups is likely to be due to the intervention. A computer-generated number sequence is one example of an appropriate randomisation method.

- The group to which the patient has been allocated must be concealed from the clinician/researcher until the patient has been accepted into the trial. This is often referred to as allocation concealment and is an important factor in reducing bias. If the clinician believes that the patient may benefit from the treatment, and realises that the patient is due to be allocated to the control group, he or she may consciously or subconsciously dissuade the patient from participating in the trial. Ideally, randomisation should be carried out by someone removed from the project, with numbers being placed in sealed, opaque envelopes. Methods based on criteria such as date of birth are not recommended as clinicians are able to work out from the date of birth and the allocation sequence which group the patient is to be allocated to.

- Demographic and health status details for the two groups are of interest. Significant differences between the two groups, for example differences in age, co-morbid conditions, gender or disease severity, could potentially affect the results of the study. The groups should ideally be similar, on average, for any variables that are likely to influence outcome. Similarity between groups is not always achieved by randomisation, even where the methods of randomisation are adequate.

- It is helpful if the intervention is described in sufficient detail to allow clinicians to reproduce it in their own setting. In addition,

Table 4.2 Quality appraisal checklist

	Criteria	Quality appraisal question	Worked example
Design	Comparative/ prospective, ideally randomised, controlled trial	Are outcomes in two or more randomly selected groups compared?	Yes Study compares children admitted with a diagnosis of acute asthma in two groups randomly allocated to receive either usual care or a specialist nurse-led discharge package
Sample	Random allocation	Are the patients randomly allocated to the groups in the study?	Yes The groups were randomly allocated in blocks of 10 using sealed envelopes to receive a structured discharge interview or standard care
	Concealment of randomisation until allocation occurs	Was allocation to the control or intervention group concealed from the patient, investigator and clinician until patient had been accepted into trial?	Yes Randomisation was held in sealed envelopes until consent had been obtained
	Baseline group comparability	Are the characteristics of both groups in the sample described and do they match on characteristics likely to affect the outcome?	Yes The baseline characteristics of the two groups are similar in terms of age, length of stay in hospital, inpatient treatment, previous attendance at A&E, and emergency consultations with a general practitioner
Measures	Intervention and outcomes clearly specified	What is the intervention/action under investigation?	The structured discharge interview included information on asthma, risk factor avoidance and drugs and devices, plus a self-management plan covering use of preventers and relievers, adjusted to symptoms and peak flow. A booklet about asthma

	What outcomes are specified?	with information on asthma organisations was also provided. Standard care involved variable amounts of information, some demonstration of device technique but few written self-management plans The main outcome measure was the rate of admission for children in the study at 6 months. Asthma symptoms, attendance without readmission, GP consultation rates and days lost from school were also measured
Researcher	Clinician/assessor/ patient masked (blinded) as to which group the patient has been allocated	Did the participants, investigators, clinicians know which groups the patients were in?	No Patients and care givers had to know they were engaged in the discharge package. However, the person making the decision as to whether to readmit children would be unlikely to be aware whether the children and their families had previously received the structured discharge package
Data	All entrants adequately accounted for at the end of the study	Was data analysis carried out using all the people who entered in the study?	Yes For the primary outcome measure at 6 month
Collection and analysis	Analysis carried out on an intention to treat basis	Were children analysed in the groups to which they were randomised?	Yes For the primary outcome measure at 6 months

the primary outcome in which the investigators would expect to see a clinically important difference should be given, along with details of how the outcome is to be measured. Measurement tools tested outside of the study and found to measure what they purport to measure, inspire more confidence than measurement tools that have not been validated.

■ Keeping patients, clinicians and researchers 'blinded' as to whether a patient is in the treatment or control group is a useful way of minimising bias. Patients who know that they are in the control group may feel that they have received substandard care and may, as a result, alter their behaviour. Similarly clinicians may consciously or subconsciously take compensatory measures for patients who are in the control group (for example by offering alternate therapies or additional support etc.). Any difference in the treatment effects between the two groups may be due to this additional attention rather than the intervention. The researcher may have preconceived ideas about the treatment and, where the outcomes of interest are fairly subjective, these preconceptions may influence the way that the researcher interprets and analyses the data. Clearly blinding is not possible in all studies, but attempts should be made to blind one (single-blind) or all (double-blind/treble-blind) of the above groups of people.

■ People drop out of studies for all sorts of reasons: death, relocation to another geographical area, treatment found to be too unpleasant, etc. It is important that the researcher tries to identify whether the reasons relate to the outcomes of interest. The analysis should be done on an 'intention to treat basis': patients are analysed in the groups to which they were randomised regardless of whether they swap from the intervention arm of the trial to the control arm or vice versa. If participants in the treatment group stop taking a drug because it makes them feel worse, and are then included in the control group, the drug may appear to be more effective than it really is due to exclusion of those patients with poor outcomes from the treatment group.

The quality assessment bottom line

This study met most of the quality criteria. The main exception is the lack of blinding, however this is a common feature of studies of non-pharmaceutical interventions as it can be difficult or impossible to conceal from the patient and the clinician what is being done. It is however often possible to blind the individual who is measuring or assessing the outcome. In this case, the primary outcome, readmission to hospital within 6 months after discharge, is an objective measure and is therefore not open to misinterpretation by the investigator. In addition the investigator would almost certainly not be responsible for deciding which children required readmission. We can conclude that the difference between the outcomes in the two groups was unlikely to be subject to bias (for the criteria examined), which suggests that we can trust the results of this study.

Worked example 4.2: Assessing the quality of a study that asks a question about whether a particular diagnostic test or method of assessment works

Scenario

Thomas Davies is a 45-year-old man has been referred to the practice nurses by his general practitioner who is 'fed up' with seeing him when there is 'nothing wrong with him'. You notice from his records that Mr Davies has been registered with the practice for 5 years. He hardly ever visited the practice until the last 3 months and since then he seems to have visited nearly every week. During your interview Mr Davies tells you that he lost his job as a supervisor in a warehouse 6 months ago and has been unable to find work since. When you question him further he tells you that he has never had any mental health problems, but during the last month he says that he has felt really down. He also feels that he has little interest in anything, so much so that some days he just sits in his armchair all day unless his wife 'nags him, to get out from under her feet'. From the information Mr Davies provides you think he might have clinical depression. You wonder how accurately a patient's self-reported loss of interest and 'feeling down' diagnoses clinical depression.

Your clinical practice question

In patients with clinical depression how accurately does patient response to questions about feeling down or depressed and loss of interest diagnose clinical depression?

Finding the evidence

You phone the local hospital library and give them your question to run a systematic search for you. They phone you a few days later and tell you that they have found the following article that they think will be useful:

> Whooley MA, Avins A, Miranda J, Browner WS 1997 Case-finding instruments for depression: two questions are as good as many. Journal of General Internal Medicine 12: 439–445

The paper reports the results of a cross-sectional study of 536 people attending a primary care setting in the USA. The study assesses the accuracy of asking just two questions (about feeling down and about loss of interest during the past month) compared with using a longer questionnaire (the National Institute of Mental Health Quick Diagnostic Interview Schedule (QDIS-III-R)) in diagnosing clinical depression.

What is the quality of the study

Table 4.3 shows a worked example of the critical appraisal for the paper referenced above that applies the quality criteria for cross-sectional studies given in Figure 4.2. The quality criteria have been adapted from the JAMA guidelines on critical appraisal (Jaeschke et al 1994). A brief explanation of why the criteria are important is provided below, but readers are referred to the JAMA guidelines for additional information.

Relevance of criteria in Table 4.3

■ An appropriate spectrum of patients (i.e. patients with mild, moderate and severe forms of the condition) should ideally be included in the study, with details of the proportions of each of these groups given. A test may be able to identify people who are severely ill, but not those with a mild form of the condition. Ideally, a consecutive set of participants who fulfil the inclusion criteria should be tested. This ensures that individuals are not inappropriately 'selected out' of the study, thereby affecting the results and conclusions of the study.

Table 4.3 Assessing the quality of a study about whether a particular test or method of assessment works

	Criteria	Quality appraisal question	Worked example
Design	Cross-sectional/comparative	Are the two methods of assessment being compared in the same patients?	Yes Patients (with and without depression) were assessed using just two questions and they were also assessed using the National Institute of Mental Health Quick Diagnostic Interview Schedule (QDIS-III-R) by trained graduate students
Sample	Appropriate spectrum of subjects	What categories of participant were included in the study?	590 consecutive patients (74 declined, 6 excluded due to blindness, 5 due to delusion/intoxication). Exclusion criteria: Patients with concurrent mania or schizophrenia (found on QDIS) were excluded from the analysis (from the 590, 47 excluded, 7 missing data). Patients were from the Urgent Care clinic in San Francisco, veterans, mean age 53, 97% male, 55% white, 8% homeless, 71% unemployed, 40% separated/divorced, 27% married. The prevalence of depression in this group was 18%
Measures	New test compared against a reference standard	What is the test/tool being compared against?	The reference standard was the National Institute of Mental Health Quick Diagnostic Interview Schedule (QDIS-III-R), administered by trained graduate students. For the purposes of the study a positive result on QDIS means that the patient really does have depression. A 20 minute face-to-face interview with a trained person is a very accurate way of diagnosing depression and this study looks at how much accuracy is lost if only two questions are asked compared to this 'exceptional practice' way of diagnosing depression

(contd.)

Table 4.3 (Contd.)

	Criteria	Quality appraisal question	Worked example
Researcher	Assessor blinded to the results of the reference standard	Did the assessors know results from the reference standard when using the test measure?	No Subjects completed the 'two questions' instrument themselves and the students were blind to their answer whilst carrying out the other diagnostic interview tests. The students had no way of knowing whether subjects had been diagnosed with clinical depression on the 'two questions' test
Data collection	New and reference standard test on all participants	Did all participants receive both new and reference standard test?	Yes
Data analysis	Intra and inter observer reliability established	Was the reliability of observer's assessment checked and, where there was more than one observer, was there consistency between the observers?	QDIS has demonstrated good test–retest reliability ($\kappa = 0.76$). Average interrater reliability for all three interviewers is reported as excellent ($\kappa = 0.88$)

- The 'new' test should be compared against the method that is currently regarded as 'the best' (i.e. the reference standard) and both tests should be applied in all participants.

- It is recommended that the clinician or investigator is 'blinded' to the results of the test that is carried out first. If the clinician suspects from the initial test that the patient does not have the disease in question, he or she may decide to avoid subjecting the patient to the second test.

- Reliability (repeatability) of a test needs to be considered: the results of tests carried out by different individuals or by the same individual at different times should remain unchanged, provided the true underlying variable that is being measured remains the same. In tests that are not repeatable, it is difficult to know whether a true measurement is being obtained.

The quality assessment bottom line

This study appears to meet the quality assessment criteria, therefore we can trust the results.

Worked example 4.3: Assessing the quality of a study that asks questions about finding out the likely pattern and/or outcome of a particular health problem/disease

Scenario

Florence Barrett, a 33-year-old mother of two, has stopped by the doctor's surgery on her way to work to collect a repeat prescription for oral contraception. You look in her case notes and notice that she has not had a pill review check this year and you invite her to return for a review the following week. You also ask her whether she is still smoking and she tells you that she smokes between 25 and 30 cigarettes per day. You note from her records that she has been using oral contraception for the last 10 years since the birth of her second child. You recall reading something about there being a higher risk of myocardial infarction (MI) in pill users who smoke and decide that before her visit you will investigate the following clinical question.

Your clinical question

Are women who smoke and take oral contraception at higher risk of MI than women who smoke but use other forms of contraception?

Finding the evidence

You begin a search on PubMed (MEDLINE via the internet) using the 'clinical queries' function and, selecting the prognosis filter, enter the terms 'myocardial infarction AND oral contraception'. Twenty citations are identified, the first of which is:

> Burkman RT 2000 Cardiovascular issues with oral contraceptives: evidence-based medicine. International Journal of Fertility and Women's Medicine 45(2): 166–174

This is a review article but does not meet the criteria of a systematic review. Neither does it provide raw data. One of the references cited is:

> Mant J, Painter R, Vessey M 1998 Risk of myocardial infarction, angina, and stroke in users of oral contraceptives: an updated analysis of a cohort study. British Journal of Obstetrics and Gynaecology 105: 890–896

The paper reports the results of a cohort study involving 17 032 women using contraception who were followed up for 20–26 years. One of the outcome measures used is the rate of MI. This is compared in women who had used oral contraception and those that had not. Subgroup analysis compares the rate of MI in women who smoke and use oral contraception and women who smoke and do not use oral contraception.

What is the quality of the study

Table 4.4 shows a worked example of the critical appraisal for the paper referenced above that uses the quality criteria given in Figure 4.2. The quality criteria have been adapted from the JAMA guidelines on critical appraisal (Laupacis et al 1994). A brief explanation of why the criteria are important is provided below, but readers are referred to the JAMA guidelines for a more detailed discussion.

Relevance of criteria in Table 4.4

- It is important that the participants in the study truly have the disorder of interest, and that they are entering the study at a

Table 4.4 Assessing the quality of a study about the likely pattern or outcome of a particular health problem or disease

	Criteria	Quality appraisal question	Worked example
Design	Longitudinal cohort study	Was a group of subjects followed up prospectively over a period of time?	Yes A cohort of 17 032 women who used contraception were recruited when they were between the ages of 25 and 39 years and followed up for between 20 and 26 years
Sample	Clearly defined, representative, assembled at a similar point	Was a defined, representative sample of patients assembled at a common (usually early) point in the course of their life and/or disease?	Yes 17 032 British, Caucasian, married women, who used contraception and were aged between 25 and 35 were recruited from 17 large family planning clinics in England and Scotland
Measures	Appropriate end points	Were appropriate end points specified in advance of the study?	Yes The outcome measures used were occurrence of angina, myocardial infarction or stroke that was associated with either hospital admission, referral to hospital or death
Researcher	No dependent relationship between subject and investigator	What is the researcher/investigator's relation to those being investigated?	The study investigators were academic staff at the University of Oxford. The study was not funded by any manufacturers of contraception

(contd.)

Table 4.4 (Contd.)

	Criteria	Quality appraisal question	Worked example
Data collection	Follow-up of adequate duration	Were the patients followed up for long enough?	Yes 17 032 women were enrolled to the study between 1968 and 1974. All women were followed up until age 45. At age 45, 15 292 women were still participating in the study. At age 45 the cohort was divided into three groups 1. Never used oral contraception (n = 5881) 2. Used oral contraception for 8 or more years 3. Remainder Only those women who had never used the oral contraceptive pill or had used the oral contraceptive pill for eight or more years were followed up after the age of 45
	All cases accounted for at end of study	Were end points given for all participants?	No End measurements were not obtained in women who dropped out of the study. Reasons for their withdrawal are not always given
Data analysis	Effects of potential confounders accounted for	Does the data analysis take into consideration the effect of any potentially confounding variables	Yes Event rates were adjusted for relevant potential confounders: age, social class, smoking, obesity and parity. In addition, the analysis was carried out twice, the second time excluding women with risk factors for a cardiovascular event (because they were less likely to be prescribed oral contraception)

N.B. These questions are specifically for the critical appraisal of cohort studies.

common point in the course of their disease. In a study aiming to identify the risk of renal disease in people with diabetes for example, if some of the participants already have undiagnosed mild kidney damage at the start of the study, it could influence the results in a negative way.

- Length of follow-up should be adequate for all possible outcomes (especially negative outcomes) to become manifest. If participants, for example people who have smoked 20 or more cigarettes a day for 1 year, are followed up for 4 years to establish risk of lung cancer, the conclusions of the study are likely to be different than if followed up for 15 years.

- People are inevitably lost to follow-up, and the reasons for this should be explored. If participants are lost to follow-up through death, rather than because they feel better, and this information is known to the researcher, he or she can take this into consideration when presenting the results.

- Outcome measurement can be a source of bias especially where the outcome is a subjective one, for example quality of life. The outcome should therefore be clearly defined in advance. In addition, where outcome measurement requires a degree of judgement, the person taking the measurement or doing the assessment should be blind to the patient's condition.

- When observing health outcomes over time, it is important to take account of the factors or variables that can affect health. In longitudinal studies, time itself acts as a confounding variable. As people get older they develop more illness regardless of any other factors. The effect of such confounding variables can be taken into account in the process of data analysis.

The quality assessment bottom line

The only area in which the quality of the study is questionable is in respect of the number of women who were lost to follow-up. The loss of patients is often unavoidable in large-scale longitudinal studies such as this one. From our point of view we are concerned about the effect this loss of patients may have on the validity of the conclusions made in the study. In all, 1740 women were lost to follow-up which is approximately 10% of the original sample. Is this too many? One way to decide is to use the '5 and 20' rule. Fewer than 5% loss probably leads to little bias, greater than 20% loss seriously threatens validity (Sackett et al 2000).

A second approach is to ask a series of 'what if?' questions known as sensitivity analysis. We can use different combinations of 'what if' scenarios to examine the possible effects of adding the missing cases back into the data analysis. The key thing here is to consider whether the cases lost to follow-up would have a different pattern of outcomes to those who remained. For our particular clinical question we would ask ourselves the question of whether the heavy smoking, oral contraception users who dropped out were any more likely to have an adverse outcome than those who remained.

Critical appraisal in practice

The critical appraisal tools given above are designed to help develop skills and knowledge of critical appraisal. Other tools produced by different organisations are available (see the 'Netting the evidence' website for more information: details are available on page 112).

Critical appraisal gets easier with practice and people quickly become adept at recognising whether they will be able to use a paper or not. Answers to the questions outlined in Tables 4.2–4.4 are often included in the abstract and methodology sections. If not, there is a high probability they are not there at all and so it may not be worth bothering to look at the rest of the paper.

It is important to remember that research is a real world process. This means that researchers are often forced to compromise on certain aspects of the research and to modify the study design for lots of legitimate reasons. There is no such thing as a perfect research study. Similarly it is also important to recognise that research is done on samples of a population who will never be identical to patients attending a clinic, the patients in a ward, etc. It is unrealistic to search for perfect research studies where the study population exactly matches a patient group. People who are new to critical appraisal may feel that no research is good enough. The trick is to identify studies that can be applied to a specific clinical context where the design is good enough for the results to be trusted.

The tools in this chapter contain the basic questions necessary for assessing the quality of research studies in the practice environment. More sophisticated critical appraisal tools and techniques are available for people who are becoming more experienced or are doing critical appraisal on questions not covered in this chapter (for example, those published as a series in the Journal of the American Medical Association, the so called JAMA guides). Details of where to find these can also be found at the 'Netting the evidence' website.

If the study is good enough to use and can be applied in the clinical setting of interest, the next step is to work out what to do about it. If a change in practice is required, how should that change be brought about? Simply telling colleagues that the evidence says they should be doing B rather than A has been demonstrated to be a rather ineffective change method (NHS CRD 1999). Methods for increasing the chance of successfully changing practice are discussed in Chapters 9 and 10.

Presenting the results of critical appraisal to colleagues in a systematic way, which makes explicit the process that was used to come to these conclusions, is an important part of preparing for change. The critical appraisal tools used above provide a method for generating a summary of a study. Another way of doing this is to use CATs or critically appraised topics, which are one-page summaries of research papers. These were developed by the Centre for Evidence Based Medicine in Oxford and examples of completed CATs can be accessed via their website (http://cebm.jr2.ox.ac.uk). They also produce CATmaker software, which is a computer program that can be used to make CATs. Raw data from the study can be entered into the program which will calculate some useful numbers for summarising the results in terms of effects on individual patients, e.g. the number needed to treat (NNT). This is discussed in more detail in Chapter 5.

Summary

This chapter has established why critical appraisal is necessary and important for evidence-based practice. The principles of research design and method underpinning the use of quality criteria to assess studies have been outlined. Critical appraisal for evidence-based practice is a three-part process comprising assessment of the quality of the study, assessment of the applicability of the study and interpretation of the study results for the individual patient.

This chapter has focused on the assessment of the quality of a study and provided practical examples of how this can be done for three different types of clinical question that require the use of different research designs. Scenario 4.1 led to a clinical question on the effectiveness of nurse-led educational interventions in families of children with asthma. The most appropriate research design for this question (in the absence of a systematic review) is an RCT. Table 4.2 gives an example of the assessment of the quality of a published RCT on this topic.

Scenario 4.2 leads to a clinical question about whether patients' self-reported feelings predict clinical depression. The most appropriate study design for this question is a cross-sectional study. Table 4.3 gives an example of the assessment of the quality of a published cross-sectional study on this topic. Scenario 4.3 generates a clinical question about whether users of oral contraception are at greater risk of MI. The most appropriate study design for this question is a longitudinal study. Table 4.4 gives an example of the assessment of quality of a published longitudinal study that addresses this question.

Acknowledgement

We would like to thank Karen Gibb, Elizabeth Pickering and Florence Sharkey for reading and providing comments on drafts of this chapter.

References

Blaikie N 2000 Designing social research. Cambridge: Polity Press

Black N 1990 Why we need observational studies to evaluate the effectiveness of health care. British Medical Journal 301: 575–580

Castledine G 1997 Barriers to evidence-based nursing care. British Journal of Nursing 6(18): 1077

Cook TD, Campbell DT 1979 Quasi-experimentation: design and analysis issues in field settings. Chicago: Rand McNally

Guyatt G, Sackett D, Cook D 1993 Users' guides to the medical literature II. How to use an article about therapy or prevention. A. Are the results of the study valid? Evidence-Based Medicine Working Group. Journal of the American Medical Association 270: 2598–2601

Jaeschke R, Guyatt G, Sackett D for the Evidence Based Medicine Working Group 1994 Users' guides to the medical literature. III. How to use an article about a diagnostic test: A. Are the results of the study valid? Journal of the American Medical Association 271: 389–391

Laupacis A, Wells G, Richardson S, Tugwell P 1994 Users' guides to the medical literature. V. How to use an article about prognosis. Journal of the American Medical Association 272: 234–237

McKee M, Britton A, Black N, McPherson K, Sanderson C, Bain C 1998 Choosing between randomised and non-randomised studies. In: Black N, Brazier J, Fitzpatrick R, Reeves B (eds) Health service research methods: a guide to best practice. London: BMJ Publications, pp 61–72

McPherson K 1994 The Cochrane Lecture: The best and the enemy of the good: randomized controlled trials, uncertainty and assessing the role of patient choice in medical decision making. Journal of Epidemiology and Community Health 4(48): 6–15

Maggs C 1997 Research and the nursing agenda: confronting what we believe nursing to be. Nursing Times Research 12(5): 321–322

Mant J 1999a Studies assessing diagnostic tests. In: Dawes M, Davies P, Gray A, Mant J, Seers J, Snowball R (eds) Evidence-based practice: a primer for health care professionals. London: Churchill Livingstone, pp 59–69

Mant J 1999b Case control studies. In: Dawes M, Davies P, Gray A, Mant J, Seers J, Snowball R (eds) Evidence-based practice: a primer for health care professionals. London: Churchill Livingstone, pp 73–85

*Mant J, Painter R, Vessey M 1998 Risk of myocardial infarction, angina, and stroke in users of oral contraceptives: an updated analysis of a cohort study. British Journal of Obstetrics and Gynaecology 105; 890–896

Moore A, McQuay H 2000 Bias. Bandolier 7(10): 1–5

Mulrow C 1994 The rationale for systematic reviews. British Medical Journal 309: 597–599

NHS CRD (NHS Centre for Reviews and Dissemination) 1999 Getting evidence into practice. Effective Health Care 5(1)

Peto R 1993 Large scale randomized evidence: large simple trials and overview trials. Annals of the New York Academy of Science 703: 314–340

Sackett D, Strauss S, Scott Richardson W, Rosenberg W, Haynes R 2000 Evidence-based medicine: how to practice and teach evidence-based medicine, 2nd edn. Edinburgh: Churchill Livingstone

Shultz KF, Chalmers I, Hayes RJ, Altman DG 1995 Empirical evidence of bias: Dimensions of methodological quality associated with estimates of treatment effects in controlled trials. Journal of the American Medical Association 273: 408–412

*Wesseldine LJ, McCarthy P, Silverman M 1999 Structured discharge procedure for children admitted to hospital with acute asthma: a randomised con-

*Papers used for critical appraisal examples.

trolled trial of nursing practice. Archives of Disease in Childhood 80: 110–114

Whooley MA, Avins A, Miranda J, Browner WS 1997 Case-finding instruments for depression: Two questions are as good as many. Journal of General Internal Medicine 12: 439–445

Further reading

Internet resources

There are numerous websites that contain materials for critical appraisal. However these sites often change their website address and new sites are opening up all the time. We have therefore provided you with the address for the most comprehensive and up-to-date information about evidence-based practice on the web, 'Netting the evidence'. This site was established and is maintained by Andrew Booth at Sheffield University.
http://www.shef.ac.uk/~scharr/ir/netting/

Books

Crombie I K 1996 The pocket guide to critical appraisal. London: BMJ Publishing

Greenhalgh T 1997 How to read a paper. London: BMJ Publishing

Ogier M E 1998 Reading research – how to make research more approachable, 2nd edn. London: Baillière Tindall

Sackett D, Strauss S, Scott Richardson W, Rosenberg W, Haynes R 2000 Evidence-based medicine: How to practice and teach evidence-based medicine, 2nd edn. Edinburgh: Churchill Livingstone

Journal articles

Cullum N 1999 Finding and appraising cohort studies. Nursing Times Learning Curve 3(7): 8–10

Nelson EA 1999 Randomised controlled trials: questions for valid evidence. Nursing Times Learning Curve 3(5): 6–8

Nelson EA 1999 Questions for surveys. Nursing Times Learning Curve 3(8): 5–7

Roberts J, DiCenso A 1999 Identifying the best research design to fit the question. Part 1: quantitative designs. Evidence-Based Nursing 2(1): 4–6

Thompson C 1999 If you could just provide me with a sample: examining sampling in qualitative and quantitative research papers. Evidence-Based Nursing 2(3): 68–70

Thompson C 1999 Questioning evidence. Nursing Times Learning Curve 3(4): 4–6

Thompson C, Cullum N 1999 Examining evidence: an overview. Nursing Times Learning Curve 3(1): 7–9

5

Critical appraisal 2: can the evidence be applied in your context?

Mark Newman and Tony Roberts

Key points

- How to decide whether the results of a study can be applied to your patients/context
- Using confidence intervals instead of '*p*-values'
- Developing a clinically useful interpretation of study results:
  - Interpreting results from a study about the effectiveness of therapies: calculating the number needed to treat (NNT)
  - Interpreting results from a study about whether or not a diagnostic test or assessment 'works': calculating likelihood ratios, pre and post test odds
  - Interpreting results from a study about prognosis or harm: calculating the number needed to harm (NNH).

Introduction

In Chapter 4 the need for research users to critically appraise published research was established. The three aspects of critical appraisal were outlined (Figure 5.1) and the methods used to assess the quality of studies examined. This chapter describes in detail the skills and knowledge that are required for the other two aspects of the critical appraisal process. The first section will discuss how to decide whether the results from a study can be applied to your patients and/or in your workplace. The second section will demonstrate how you can translate the results given for a study sample into clinically meaningful results for an individual patient. The three scenarios developed in Chapter 4, and their respective pieces of evidence, will be used to illustrate this process.

Deciding whether the results can be applied in your setting

This section is concerned with developing the skills and knowledge necessary for deciding whether it is appropriate to apply the findings of a research project to a specific patient (Figure 5.1). Health-related research takes place all over the world, in settings that may be very different from the one in which your patients are found. In addition, research is carried out on samples from the wider population. The context in which you practise and/or the context of each patient's consultation are to some degree unique. Health care practitioners need to be able to decide whether the results obtained in a study that used a particular sample can be applied to their patient/context, which may in some respects be different.

Seek to include not exclude studies

The patients and settings used in a research study will never be identical to yours. When considering the issue of applicability it is more useful to ask the question 'are my patients/setting so different that results will not apply?', than to ask 'are these patients exactly the same age, gender, etc. as the patients in my clinic/ward?' If there are differences, it is useful to ask how these differences might affect

Figure 5.1 **Aspects of the critical appraisal process. 2: Assessing applicability**

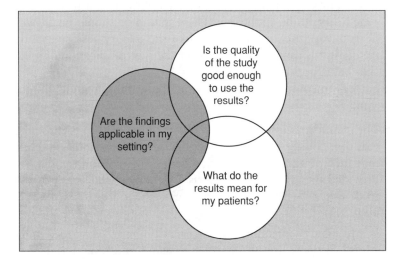

the results. If the differences would only change the size or extent of the effect of the treatment, rather than changing the effect from one of benefit to one of harm, then it may be possible to adjust the result to reflect the impact in your patients. For example, participants enrolled in research studies tend to be fitter than patients in usual practice conditions. This could mean that a different outcome will occur should the therapy/test be used on a very sick patient. (However, it may also mean that the patients will simply derive greater benefits than those in the study: sick patients are more likely to benefit more from treatments.) These issues are illustrated in the discussions of the interpretations of the results for each scenario under the heading 'The clinical bottom line'.

Questions for assessing applicability and screening

In practice there is considerable overlap between the process of assessing the quality of a study (as described in Chapter 4) and the process of assessing its applicability. To a certain extent both processes are carried out simultaneously. On the basis that it is usually easier to assess applicability, questions relating to this aspect of critical appraisal can be used as a form of screening as illustrated in Figure 5.2. If the results of a study cannot be applied in your situation, then there is no need to read further or to continue with the other aspects of the critical appraisal process.

A series of questions is used to ascertain whether the patients and/or context in a particular study are too dissimilar to your own for the results to be applicable. These questions should be answerable from the research report. Unlike the quality assessment, the same questions can be used whatever the type of question or study design being appraised.

Factors to consider when assessing applicability include the following:

- The characteristics of the participants in the study, i.e. those factors that could potentially affect the outcomes of interest. These may include age, co-morbidity, severity of condition, gender, etc. Provided the relevant characteristics are provided, it is possible to determine whether the study participants are similar to your own.

- Is it feasible to introduce the intervention or test described in the study? Suppose the results of a research study undertaken to look at the care of patients with stroke suggest that patient outcomes are better when they are looked after in a specialist unit (i.e. one that requires certain types of equipment and staff with specialist training) rather than in a general ward. Such a change may not be possible on your unit. This does not mean that you should give up all together (the issue should perhaps be referred to your unit manager), however it does mean that you will need to look at other aspects of stroke management that are within the capacity of your team to deliver.

■ When thinking of the costs and benefits of the intervention or test, think beyond purely financial terms. In most situations

Figure 5.2 Screening a research study for applicability

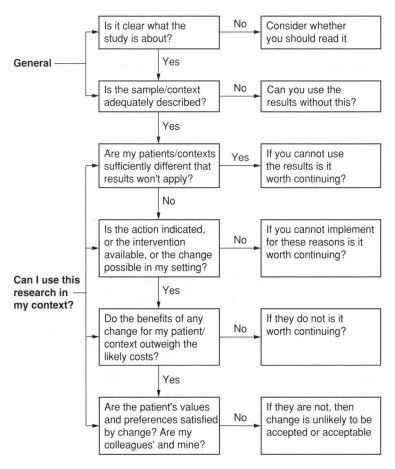

doing something new or in a different way will involve stopping doing something else. The costs of 'stopping' need to be weighed up against the benefits of the proposed change. Where the costs are perceived by the patient and/or staff as being too high, the proposed change is unlikely to be accepted.

■ Patient preference needs to be taken into account. Evidence is not the only factor that informs clinical decision-making. Patients may have strong preferences for or against a particular intervention. Forcing a patient to use the intervention indicated by evidence would be unethical and may be counter-productive.

Table 5.1 lists the questions to be asked when assessing applicability and provides answers for the example of the case of Florence Barrett (see Chapter 4, Worked example 4.3, page 103). The relevant aspects of the scenario have been reproduced in Box 5.1.

What do the results of this study mean in my context/for my patients?

It is a common misperception that evidence-based practice is all about statistics. We hope that it is already clear that this is not the case. The evidence-based practice approach is that the statistical analyses carried out in a study are not the most important consideration when critically appraising a paper. Most important is the quality of the study design. If a study was well designed then there

---

> **Box 5.1 Information from the scenario in Worked example 4.3 relevant to the assessment of applicability**
>
> *Patient*: Florence Barrett, 35 years old, mother of two, used oral contraception for the last 10 years, smokes 25–30 cigarettes per day.
> *Clinical question*: Is Florence, a heavy smoker using the oral contraceptive pill, at higher risk of myocardial infarction than women who smoke but use other forms of contraception?
> *Evidence*: Mant J, Painter R, Vessey M 1998 Risk of myocardial infarction, angina, and stroke in users of oral contraceptives: an updated analysis of a cohort study. British Journal of Obstetrics and Gynaecology 105: 890–896

Table 5.1 **Questions for assessing the applicability of a study**

Question	Example: Scenario 4.3
What is the study about?	The study investigated the risk of myocardial infarction, angina and stroke in users of oral contraceptives compared with users of other methods of contraception
Who are the participants in the study (e.g. diagnosis, age, gender, occupation)?	The study included women aged 25–39 who attended 17 family planning clinics in England and Scotland. Both smokers and non-smokers were included. All women were British, married and Caucasian
In what way are our patients/contexts different?	Those study participants who smoke can be assumed to be similar to Florence Barrett
Where is the study set (country, institution)?	Participants in the study were recruited from family planning clinics in England and Scotland
Is/are the change(s) indicated possible in our setting (if not, why?)?	As this was a study about prognosis or outcomes this question is less relevant. However, if the results suggested that Florence was at greater risk of an MI if she continued to use oral contraception there are no impediments to changing the method of contraception Florence uses apart from her own preferences
What are the benefits of the change(s) indicated (to whom)?	The potential benefit to Florence is a reduction in her risk of MI. This has potential knock-on benefits for members of her family and the health services
What are the costs (financial or otherwise) of the change(s) and to whom?	Potential costs to Florence and her family include increased risk of unwanted pregnancy and increased inconvenience that other suitable methods of contraception might entail. These costs may be hidden from the view of health professionals but should not be underestimated
In what ways do the change(s) indicated meet with your patients' (or your own) values and preferences?	No information is given about Florence's preferred method of contraception. Her visit to the surgery was not prompted by a desire to change methods, suggesting she is happy enough with the oral contraceptive pill. The results about her level of risk of myocardial infarction (her overall risk can be calculated using CHD risk calculators) should be discussed with her to allow her to come to her own decision after weighing up the relative benefits and costs of any change

is a high probability that the researchers' interpretation of the results can be trusted (Sackett et al 2000). Even well done statistical analysis cannot compensate for bias caused by deficiencies in the study design.

However, once you have decided the quality of the study is good enough, and the results can be applied to your patient, the next stage is to interpret what the results of the study mean for your individual patient. This is the third aspect of critical appraisal for EBP highlighted in Figure 5.3. The way the results of research are reported can often make it difficult to interpret the results for application in daily clinical practice. One reason for this is that one of the major concerns of researchers is to establish the likelihood of their result being caused by chance. For example the proportion of children readmitted within 6 months of discharge in the study of nurse-led intervention to prevent asthma is reported as 37% in the control group versus 15% in the intervention group ($\chi^2 = 10.5$, $p < 0.001$). (Wesseldine et al 1999). χ^2 is a test which shows whether the difference in outcome between the two groups is statistically significant. A p-value <0.001 tells us that the probability of this being a chance result is less than 1 in 1000, it is unlikely that the result is due to chance. The p-value does not give any indication of the size or direction of the difference (or treat-

Figure 5.3 Aspects of the critical appraisal process.
            3: Interpreting results

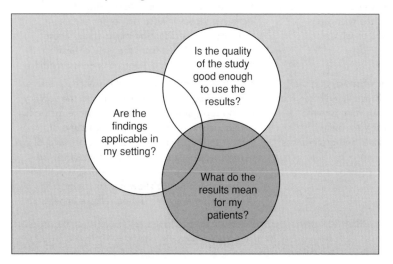

ment effect) (Gardner & Altman 1986). Therefore, it does not help you assess what the likely affect will be on your patient.

A number of more clinically meaningful measures have been developed for different types of question/study designs. One example is the number needed to treat (NNT), which is useful for interpreting results from studies about the effectiveness of a therapy or intervention (Laupacis et al 1988). NNT shows how many patients have to be given the intervention for one extra person to benefit who would not have done so if given the comparison treatment. Studies that look at whether a particular method of diagnosis or assessment works often give results as the sensitivity (proportion of people with a condition who test positive) and specificity (proportion of people without the condition who test negative) of the test. These can be converted (using likelihood ratios) into probabilities that express how likely the diagnosis is for a particular patient.

More studies are being published which use these types of measures to report their results but health care practitioners will continue to need to understand how to calculate these themselves. At first some of the calculations may seem a bit intimidating. However, despite their complexity to look at, they usually only involve some simple arithmetic that can, if necessary, be done with pencil and paper. The most effective way of learning these techniques is by working through real examples. The following sections will describe how these measures are calculated, using as examples the results given in the papers we have already critically appraised in Chapter 4.

Interpreting the results of studies about the effectiveness of a particular therapy or intervention

This section will describe how the data from a study can be used to calculate the number needed to treat (NNT). The results from the paper referenced in Worked example 4.1 (page 94) will be used (Box 5.2).

Developing a clinically meaningful result

A 2 × 2 table like the one shown in Figure 5.4 is a standard tool used for calculating clinically meaningful results and will be used in

> **Box 5.2 Information from the scenario in Worked example 4.1 relevant to an assessment of the effectiveness of an intervention**
>
> *Patient*: Sally Gibson, 11 years old with four admissions for acute asthma in previous 6 months.
>
> *EBP question*: Does a structured nurse-led discharge package result in reduced levels of readmission to hospital of children with acute asthma?
>
> *Evidence*: Wesseldine LJ, McCarthy P, Silverman M 1999 Structured discharge procedure for children admitted to hospital with acute asthma: a randomised controlled trial of nursing practice. Archives of Disease in Childhood 80: 110–114
>
> *Results reported in the study*: The abstract contains the main results which are reported as a reduction in the admission at 6 months (12 of 80 in the intervention group versus 30 of 80 in the control group), lower attendance at the A&E department (6 of 80 versus 31 of 80) and visits to the GP for problematic asthma (31 of 78 versus 72 of 77). We are told that all these results are statistically significant.

each example in this chapter. Each cell in the table contains a number and is labelled with a letter, a, b, c and d. In a comparative study participants are divided into two groups: the group which received the 'new' or experimental therapy (cells a and b) and the group

Figure 5.4 **A 2 × 2 table for interpreting results of a study on the effectiveness of an intervention with data from the study by Wesseldine and colleagues**

		Outcome: Readmission within 6 months		Totals
		Present	Absent	
Study groups	Experimental group (discharge package)	12 a	b 68	a + b 80
	Control group (usual care)	30 c	d 50	c + d 80
Totals		42 a + c	b + d 118	a + b + c + d 160

which did not (cells c and d). The presence (cells a and c) or absence (cells b and d) of the outcome of interest is reported for both groups. The letters in the cells are used in the formulae for calculating summary results like the number needed to treat (NNT) shown in Table 5.2. The numbers to go in each cell are obtained from the study results. It is often possible to calculate the numbers if they are not given. Figure 5.4 uses the results from the study conducted by Wesseldine and colleagues, the study being used in this scenario.

Calculating the number needed to treat (NNT)

The formulae for calculating the measures described in this section are given in Table 5.2. In order to calculate the NNT some other simple calculations are required. First, we need to calculate the experimental event rate (EER). This tells us the percentage of children in the structured discharge group that were readmitted within 6 months. Secondly, we need to calculate the control event rate (CER). This tells us the percentage of children in the usual care group that were readmitted within 6 months. These two figures are needed for the third step, calculating the absolute risk reduction (ARR). The ARR is needed to calculate the NNT. The NNT represents the number of patients who would have to receive the new intervention to obtain a beneficial result for one extra patient who would otherwise have not obtained that benefit. The smaller the NNT the more important the treatment effect. In this example the NNT is 5 (the figure is rounded up toward the more conservative whole number). This means that five children need to receive the structured discharge package to prevent one extra child from being readmitted who would have been readmitted if they had received standard care.

Table 5.2 **Calculating the number needed to treat (NNT)**

Step	Measure	Formulae	Example
1	Experimental event rate (EER)	a/a + b	12/12 + 68 = 15%
2	Control event rate (CER)	c/c + d	30/30 + 50 = 37%
3	Absolute risk reduction (ARR)	CER–EER	37 – 15 = 22%
4	Number needed to treat (NNT)	100/ARR	100/22 = 5 (rounded-up)

Measuring clinical importance – confidence intervals

Confidence intervals are a clinically useful way of measuring the precision of an estimate of effect size. The accepted convention is to use the 95% confidence interval. This is the range around the point estimate obtained from a study within which on 95 out of 100 occasions the true result lies. The narrower the gap between the upper and lower 95% confidence intervals the more certain we will be about the precision of the estimate. The 95% confidence intervals can be calculated for most common statistical estimates or comparisons including the ARR and the NNT (Altman 1998, Gardner & Altman 1986). For example, in the study by Wesseldine and colleagues the NNT for preventing readmission at 6 months in the sample population is 5. The 95% confidence intervals are 3 and 11 (see Box 5.3). This means that we can be 95% confident that the true NNT for this intervention lies somewhere between 3 and 11. The ARR for readmission at 6 months was 22% (see Table 5.2) with the 95% confidence intervals between 9% and 35%. This means that we can be 95% certain that the true ARR is somewhere between 9% and 35%. The method for calculating confidence intervals for the ARR and NNT is shown in Box 5.3.

Box 5.3 Calculating 95% confidence intervals for the ARR and NNT

Formula 95% CI for ARR $= +/- 1.96 \sqrt{\dfrac{EER\ (100-EER)}{a+b} + \dfrac{CER(100-CER)}{c+d}}$

Example using data from the study by Wesseldine et al (1999)

95% CI for ARR $= +/- 1.96 \sqrt{\dfrac{15\ (100-15)}{80} + \dfrac{37\ (100-37)}{80}}$

95% CI for ARR $= +/- 13\%$

Formula 95% CI for NNT= 100/upper 95% CI to 100/lower 95% CI of the ARR

Example using data from the study by Wesseldine et al (1999)

95% CI for NNT   =   100/33 to 100/9

95% CI for NNT   =   3 to 11

The same calculations can be used to look at the other outcomes presented in the paper. You can use these to practise calculating the ARRs and NNTs for accident and emergency attendance and general practitioner consultation rates.

The clinical bottom line

The clinical bottom line refers to what the results actually mean for clinical practice. The clinical bottom line for the study in this example could be described as follows. In children admitted with a diagnosis of acute asthma, a nurse-led structured discharge package including a self-management plan prevents an admission to hospital for one child for every five children who receive it. Sally Gibson, being 11 and with several admissions for acute asthma, would have been eligible for the study. There is no reason to suppose that she would not have benefited from the intervention. Despite being in an older age group (young children are at higher risk of readmission than older ones), she may be at higher risk than the average child in the study. This is supported by the fact that she has had four admissions (only three children in the control group had this many admissions). If Sally were at higher risk, the NNT to help her might be even lower than the average NNT (5) reported here. However, if the service were to routinely benefit your asthma patients a discharge procedure like the one in the study would need to be set up. You will need to think about whether colleagues can be persuaded to consider this as a possible use of any limited resources available (especially nursing time). Putting a case forward for such a service development would depend, in part, on the evidence of effectiveness for the service.

Interpreting the results of studies about whether a particular diagnostic test or method of assessment works

This section will focus on calculating and understanding some clinically useful measures for interpreting the results of studies that measure how good a test or method of assessment is at finding a target condition. These include sensitivity, specificity, positive and negative likelihood ratios and pre- and post-test probabilities. The results from the paper referenced in Working example 4.2 will be used as an example (see Chapter 4, page 99). The relevant details from the paper and scenario are given in Box 5.4.

Developing a clinically meaningful result

The results of diagnostic studies are usually reported in terms of sensitivity (the chance of having a positive result using the 'two questions' if you have depression) and specificity (the chance of having a negative result using the 'two questions' if you do not have depression). These figures are given in the example paper (Box 5.4). A high sensitivity is a useful result because the presence of a negative test result in a patient virtually rules out a positive diagnosis. In this example (sensitivity 96%), we could say that if Mr Davies answers 'No' to the two questions we can be fairly sure that he does not have depression (we would only be wrong in four patients out of 100).

A high specificity is a useful result because a positive test result in an individual patient effectively rules in a positive diagnosis. In

---

Box 5.4 Information from the scenario in Worked example 4.2 relevant to an assessment of a diagnostic test

Scenario: Thomas Davies, a 45-year-old frequent attender, visits practice nurse, unemployed, no mental health problems, self-reported 'feeling down and loss of interest'. Nurse feels that he has a 50% chance of having clinical depression (which means he has 50% chance of not having clinical depression).

Clinical question: In patients with clinical depression how accurately does patient response to questions about feeling down or depressed and loss of interest diagnose clinical depression?

Evidence: Whooley MA, Avins A, Miranda J, Browner WS 1997 Case-finding instruments for depression: two questions are as good as many. Journal of General Internal Medicine 12: 439–445

Results: A positive response to the two-item instrument had a sensitivity of 96% (95% CI 90–99%) and a specificity 57% (95% CI 53–62%).

this example (specificity 57%) if Mr Davies answers 'yes' to the two questions we could not be sure that he had clinical depression. Forty-three patients in 100 answer yes to one of the questions but do not have clinical depression. Whilst the sensitivity and specificity are useful when they are high, it is rare that both the sensitivity and specificity are both high on the same test as there is nearly always a trade-off between the two.

In addition, the performance of a test is affected by the prevalence of the condition in the underlying population. In an individual patient, this is referred to as the pre-test probability of an individual having the condition. In our scenario the nurse thought that Mr Davies had a pre-test probability of 50% of having clinical depression (which means he has 50% probability of not having clinical depression). What the nurse wants the test to do is to increase this probability to as near 100% as possible, either that he does or does not have depression. This is called the post-test probability.

In a study which tests whether a diagnostic test or assessment works, the new test is compared to an existing 'gold standard'. This is a method that is assumed to diagnose the target condition with certainty. All patients with and without the condition receive both tests. The results of the study can be reported in a 2 × 2 table. Figure 5.5 shows a 2 × 2 table complete with data from the study on the 'Two questions for depression' (Whooley et al 1997). In this study the gold standard is the score obtained using the QDIS questionnaire.

Figure 5.5 **A 2 × 2 table showing results from the 'two questions' diagnostic study**

		Target disorder: Depression as diagnosed by QDIS score		Totals
		Present	Absent	
New test: 'two questions'	Positive	93 a	b 189	a + b 282
	Negative	4 c	d 250	c + d 254
Totals		97 a + c	b + d 439	a + b + c + d 536

Calculating the difference between the pre- and post-test probability

What the nurse and Mr Davies need to know is, does answering yes or no to these two questions mean that Mr Davies does or does not have clinical depression? Technically this is the likelihood that a positive test result is a true positive and that a negative test result is a true negative. The ratio of true positive results to false positive results is known as the positive likelihood ratio. The ratio of true negative results to false negative results is known as the negative likelihood ratio. We can calculate these from the sensitivity and specificity respectively. The formulae to calculate these measures are given in Table 5.3. Using the data from the study by Whooley et al the positive likelihood ratio = 2.2. This means that an answer of yes to the 'two questions' is more than twice as likely in someone who has clinical depression than in someone who does not (i.e. to be a true positive rather than a false positive).

However, this is still not a very helpful result. The likelihood ratio of 2 in this example is only moderately positive. The question arises of twice as likely as what? If Mr Davies was very unlikely to be clinically depressed before taking the test then being twice as likely does not necessarily mean that he is clin-

Table 5.3 **Formulae for calculating useful clinical measures for answering questions about whether a particular diagnostic test or method of assessment works**

Measure	Formula	Example (Worked example 4.2 data)
Sensitivity	a/a + c	93/97 = 0.96 or 96%
Specificity	d/b + d	250/439 = 0.57 or 57%
Positive likelihood ratio	Sensitivity/100 − specificity	96/100 − 57 = 2.2
Negative likelihood ratio	100 − sensitivity/specificity	(100 − 96)/57 = 0.07
Pre-test odds	Prevalence/100 − prevalence	50/(100−50) = 1
Post-test odds	Pre-test probability × likelihood ratio	1 × 2 = 2
Post-test probability	Post-test odds/post-test odds + 1	2/(2 + 1) = 0.67 or 67%

ically depressed. The interpretation of likelihood ratios depends partly on the underlying prevalence (Mant 1999). The pre-test probability of 50 : 50, which is the same as pre-test odds of 1 : 1, can be combined with the likelihood ratio to give us the post-test odds or probability. In this example 1 : 1 can be multiplied with the likelihood ratio 2 giving post-test odds of 2 : 1 in favour of clinical depression. If, like us, you are more comfortable with probability than odds, post-test odds of 2 : 1 converts to a more useful but not diagnostic post-test probability of 67%.

Calculating post-test probability using the nomogram

Another simpler way of calculating Mr Davies' chance of having depression given a result from the 'two questions' method is to use the nomogram shown in Figure 5.6. Find 50% on the left-hand column, then find 2.2 in the middle column (the positive likelihood ratio) and read off the post-test probability on the right hand column (about 67%). This means that there is still a 33% chance that, even given a positive result using the two questions method, Mr Davies does not have depression. For a negative result, find 50% on the left-hand column again, then find 0.07 (the negative likelihood ratio) in the middle column and read off the post-test probability (about 4–5%). This means that if Mr Davies answers no to the two questions there is a 95% chance that he does not have clinical depression.

The clinical bottom line

The clinical bottom line in our example study could be as follows: Using a quick assessment tool can rule out depression in primary care settings. This allows more detailed assessment to be targeted at cases where the assessment is positive. The results of the study suggest that a negative result using the two questions method indicates that it is very unlikely that Mr Davies is clinically depressed (about a 2% chance). A positive result does not really increase our certainty in a diagnosis of clinical depression. In our scenario Mr Davies has reported both loss of interest and feeling down (he is positive for the two questions). So he may well have clinical depression. However, a more detailed assessment, perhaps by a psychologist or counsellor, may be necessary to firmly establish the correct diagnosis.

Figure 5.6 **Likelihood ratio nomogram showing interpretation of data from the study by Whooley et al (1997) applied to the scenario in Worked example 4.2 (Chapter 4, page 99). (From Sackett et al 2000 Evidence based medicine: how to practice and teach EBM, 2nd edn. Edinburgh: Churchill Livingstone, with permission.)**

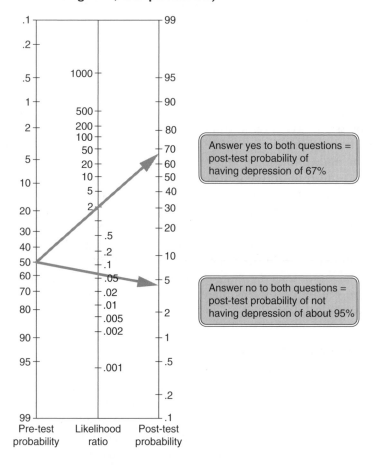

Interpreting the results of studies about prognosis or outcome of a particular condition and/or harm

If we are satisfied that the evidence from a study can be applied and is of good enough quality to use, then we need to decide if the association between exposure and outcome is sufficiently strong and convincing for us to have to do something about it. Working example 4.3 can be used to illustrate this (see Chapter 4, page 103). Relevant details from the paper and scenario are given in Box 5.5. Studies of prognosis/harm usually report results in terms of proportions or rates of events in the two groups being compared. In this scenario the result of interest is the difference between the rate of myocardial infarctions in women who smoke more than 15 cigarettes a day and use the oral contraceptive pill and women who smoke more than 15 cigarettes a day but have never used the oral contraceptive pill. For the clinical question in the scenario the results of interest can be found in the text that describes table 2 and in table 2 itself in the paper by Mant et al (1998). In this study the researchers have quite appropriately adjusted the results for other potential confounding variables such as age, parity, social class and obesity.

Box 5.5 Information from the scenario in Worked example 4.3 relevant to the assessment of association between exposure and outcome

Patient: Florence Barrett, 33 years old, mother of two, used oral contraception for the last 10 years, smokes 25–30 cigarettes per day.

Clinical question: Are women who smoke and take oral contraception at higher risk of myocardial infarction than women who smoke but use other forms of contraception?

Evidence: Mant J, Painter R, Vessey M 1998 Risk of myocardial infarction, angina, and stroke in users of oral contraceptives: an updated analysis of a cohort study. British Journal of Obstetrics and Gynaecology 105: 890–896

Results: In heavy smokers there is a fourfold increase in the risk of myocardial infarction if the oral contraceptive pill is taken, from 0.24 per 1000 women-years in heavy smokers who have never used oral contraception to 1.18 per 1000 women-years at risk in current users of oral contraception. In heavy smokers (15+) the relative risk is 4.0 for ex-users of the oral contraceptive pill, 4.2 for ever-users of the oral contraceptive pill and 4.9 for current users.

Developing a clinically meaningful result

The outcome of interest is the difference between the rate in the YES (heavy smoker, user of the oral contraceptive pill) group and the rate in the NO (heavy smoker, never used the oral contraceptive pill) group. There are several different ways in which we can interpret this difference, some of which are reported in the paper. A 2 × 2 table can be used to aid interpretation of the study results. A 2 × 2 table using the headings from the study by Mant and colleagues is given in Figure 5.7. The raw data are not reported in the paper, only the resulting rates.

Relative risk and its limitations

One of the results reported in the study by Mant et al (1998) is the relative risk (RR). Researchers often report the RR as a measure of effect size. This measures the relative difference in the percentage affected in each group. For example, where the results of a study show that the percentage affected in one group is 0.0025 and in the other 0.01 this can legitimately be presented as a fourfold difference in the relative risk between groups. However, in this example the absolute difference between the two groups is less than 1%. Depending on the question or the study, different measures will be important. For example, if the outcome is mortality a difference of 0.75% may be considered sufficient to change practice. If the outcome is benefit obtained by using a very expensive drug with unpleasant side effects, a difference of 0.75% may not be considered sufficient to change practice.

Figure 5.7 **A 2 × 2 table for prognostic/harm studies (scenario in Worked example 4.3 from Chapter 4, page 103)**

		Adverse outcome: Myocardial infarction		Rates
		Present	Absent	
Exposed to the treatment (oral contraception)	Yes: Heavy smokers, use oral contraceptives	a	b	a/(a + b) = rate in Yes group
	No: Heavy smokers, never used oral contraceptives	c	d	c/(c + d) = rate in No group

In this example the RR tells us that the rate of myocardial infarctions per 1000 women-years is 4.9 times greater amongst women who smoke heavily and use oral contraception compared with women who smoke heavily and have never used oral contraception. As a general rule of thumb in cohort studies we can say that a relative risk increase of more than 3 is unlikely to be the result of bias (Sackett et al 2000). From the results of the paper we can deduce that there is a difference in rates between the two groups and that this difference is unlikely to be the result of bias. But is the difference big enough to recommend a change of contraception method for Mrs Barrett?

Calculating the number needed to harm (NNH)

There are a number of other measures we can calculate to help Mrs Barrett make that decision. Table 5.4 shows the formulae for these calculations with completed examples using data from the study by Mant et al. In order to calculate the Number Needed to Harm (NNH) we first need to calculate the absolute risk increase (ARI). The ARI tells us the size of the difference between the two groups. The ARI in this example tells that the difference between the groups is equivalent to less than 1 event per 1000 women-years. Florence Barrett is not going to live for 1000 years so what does this result mean to her? Another way of presenting this result is to use the Number Needed to Harm. The NNH tells us the number of women who smoke heavily that would have to take oral contraception for 1 year to cause one extra myocardial infarction. In the example the NNH = 1063 (for some reason this figure is given as 1060 in the abstract of the paper by Mant et al (1998)).

Table 5.4 Formulae for calculating useful clinical measures for answering questions about prognosis/harm

Measure	Formula	Example
Relative risk (RR)	$(a/(a + b))/(c/(c + d))$	$1.18/0.24 = 0.49$
Absolute risk increase (ARI)	$(a/(a + b)) -(c/(c + d))$	$1.18 - 0.24 = 0.94$ per 1000
Number needed to harm (NNH)	$1/ARI$	$1/0.00094[a] = 1063$

[a] Rate per 1000 converted to percentage by dividing by 1000.

Clinical bottom line

The clinical bottom line for this study might be as follows. There is an increased risk of myocardial infarction in heavy smokers who use oral contraception. This increased risk is very small. A total of 1063 heavy smokers would need to take oral contraception for 1 year for one extra woman to experience a myocardial infarction. As a heavy smoker, Mrs Barrett is at greater risk of having a myocardial infarction if she continues to use oral contraception. This increase in risk is comparatively small. The benefit she might gain from switching methods of contraception is probably even smaller than the results given here suggest, as she will not return to the level of risk of a person who has never used oral contraception. The possible benefits in terms of a small reduction in risk of myocardial infarction have to be weighed up against a possibly larger increase in risk of unwanted pregnancy.

Summary

This chapter has described how you can decide whether the results of a study can be applied in your setting and how you can calculate clinically useful measures to interpret the results given in studies for your patients/setting. These two processes, combined with the process used to assess the quality of studies described in Chapter 4, make up the critical appraisal process. It is important to recognise that all three aspects of the critical appraisal process are interlinked. The quality and applicability aspects are probably the most important parts of critical appraisal to learn. Only you know the setting in which you wish to apply the results and published studies very rarely assess their own quality, whereas it is becoming more common to publish study results in clinically useful forms.

The information obtained in the process of deciding on the applicability of a study and the clinically useful measures can be combined with the quality assessment results in a critically appraised topic (CAT), which can then be shared with your colleagues and patients. However it is important to recognise that critical appraisal is only one part of the EBP process and on its own will not result in improvements in the quality of care that you might want to achieve. It is therefore important that you take equal care to learn and practise the other stages in the EBP process described in the other chapters of this manual.

Acknowledgement

We would like to thank Karen Gibb, Elizabeth Pickering amd Florence Sharkey for reading and providing comments on drafts of this chapter.

References

Altman DG 1998 Confidence intervals for the number needed to treat. British Medical Journal 317: 1309–1312

Gardner M, Altman DG 1986 Confidence intervals rather than P values: estimation rather than hypothesis testing. British Medical Journal 292: 746–750

Laupacis A, Sackett DL, Roberts RS 1988 An assessment of clinically useful measures of the consequences of treatment. New England Journal of Medicine 318(26): 1728–1733

Mant J 1999 Is this test effective? In: Dawes M, Davies P, Gray A, Mant J, Seers J, Snowball R (eds) Evidence-based practice: a primer for health care professionals. London: Churchill Livingstone, pp 133–157

*Mant J, Painter R, Vessey M 1998 Risk of myocardial infarction, angina, and stroke in users of oral contraceptives: an updated analysis of a cohort study. British Journal of Obstetrics and Gynaecology 105: 890–896

Sackett D, Strauss S, Scott Richardson W, Rosenberg W, Haynes R 2000 Evidence-based medicine: how to practice and teach evidence-based medicine, 2nd edn. Edinburgh: Churchill Livingstone

*Wesseldine LJ, McCarthy P, Silverman M 1999 Structured discharge procedure for children admitted to hospital with acute asthma: a randomised controlled trial of nursing practice. Archives of Disease in Childhood 80: 110–114

*Whooley MA, Avins A, Miranda J, Browner WS 1997 Case-finding instruments for depression: two questions are as good as many. Journal of General Internal Medicine 12: 439–445

Further reading

See Chapter 4, page 112

---

*Papers used for critical appraisal examples.

6

Qualitative methods and evidence-based practice

Andrea Litva and Ann Jacoby

Key points

- Describe the nature of qualitative inquiry
- Explain the different types of qualitative data collection
- Understand how to appraise qualitative research
- Understand how qualitative research can inform clinical practice.

Introduction

There is a growing awareness amongst medical disciplines of the need to extend the boundaries in the types of research used to contribute to the practice of evidence-based medicine (Black 1994, Popay & Williams 1998, Pope & Mays 1995). Muir Gray (1997) asserts that the practice of evidence-based medicine requires information obtained using a range of research methods, thus moving beyond the discipline of clinical epidemiology which currently underpins it (Barbour 2000, Green & Britten 1998). This requires the practitioner to engage with qualitative methods, which are best suited to investigating the beliefs, attitudes and preferences of practitioners and patients, and so can aid understanding of how evidence is turned into practice.

This chapter begins with an outline of the nature of qualitative research, providing a brief summary of different types of research methods used. We then describe the various ways in which the quality of research using qualitative methods can be assessed. The chapter concludes by exploring how a qualitative approach can inform clinical practice. This includes both the production and application of clinical evidence. Throughout the chapter, examples of qualitative studies are used to demonstrate how different methods can produce findings to inform clinical practice.

What is qualitative research?

A central feature of qualitative research is that it does not seek to produce quantified answers to research questions (Pope & Mays 1995). The goal of qualitative research is to produce insights on the social world, within natural settings by giving emphasis to the meanings, experiences, practices and views of those involved. Qualitative research is non-positivistic, meaning that insights are 'interpreted' rather than 'uncovered'. 'Truth' is considered to be relative to its context, not absolute. It may appear in the first instance that qualitative research shares certain qualities with personal anecdotes or journalism, but it is vastly different in practice. While stories are told for their dramatic or other informative qualities, they are done so without analysis or critical evaluation. Whether we believe these stories is usually based upon who is telling them. In contrast, good qualitative research requires such elements as explicit sampling strategies and detailed explanations of how data have been systematically collected and analysed to give the reader confidence in the conclusions drawn. In this section, the features that are characteristic of all qualitative research are described. While they can be found in all examples of qualitative research, it is important to recognise that there can be great variability in practice, in relation to each of the characteristics.

Naturalistic inquiry

There is no standard approach in qualitative research (Silverman 1993). However, Marshal & Rossman (1989) have demonstrated that the various strands in qualitative research have in common a commitment to naturally occurring data or naturalistic inquiry – that is, to studying phenomena within their natural setting rather than within an artificial or controlled one. Naturalistic inquiry has been described by Guba (1981) as a 'discovery-oriented' approach that minimises investigator manipulation of the study setting and places no prior constraint on what the outcomes will be. Qualitative research is committed to understanding real world situations as they unfold, from the point of view of the people who live in these worlds. This involves entering their worlds and trying to see things from their point of view. The researcher makes no attempt to manipulate the research setting, but at the same time is aware of the impact they can have upon it. This is different from experimental research, where the investigator usually attempts to control study conditions by manipulating, changing or holding constant external influences, so that a limited set of measurable outcome variables are produced.

Emphasis on the meanings, views, experiences and practices of the informants

Bryman (1988) states that the profound commitment to viewing any phenomenon from the perspective of the people being studied is one of the most fundamental features of any qualitative inquiry. Silverman (1993) broadens this point to include a focus upon uncovering the behaviours or practices of informants. The emphasis is upon making sense of settings and human actions by letting the researcher get as close to the informants as possible. In doing so, the researcher, in effect, becomes the research instrument and the quality of the research is greatly dependent upon the researchers' ability to develop rapport with informants, collect data systematically and interpret them (Guba & Lincoln 1981). In qualitative research, there is clear acknowledgement that observer bias cannot be avoided. Instead, open disclosure of preconceptions and assumptions that can influence data collection and analysis becomes part of the conduct of inquiry. It is therefore not uncommon for a qualitative researcher to provide a brief account of their personal bias – disclosure – in order to encourage informants' voices to be the ones that ultimately emerge.

An inductive process

Qualitative research is inductive as opposed to deductive: the research proceeds from the ground up. It begins with observations of phenomena, constructs, explanations or understandings, building towards generating theories. In some instances, qualitative researchers opt for an open and unstructured strategy, refusing to impose pre-formulated theoretical frameworks and concepts in advance of the study (Bryman 1988, Glaser & Strauss 1967). Alternatively, qualitative research may be influenced by a particular theory that informs the questions asked and of whom (e.g. feminist research), but still allows data to emerge in such a way as to explore the extent to which the theoretical framework is supported by the research findings.

Context and holism

Central to qualitative research is the importance of context and understanding phenomena holistically. Rather than seeking to isolate and manipulate variables, qualitative research seeks to study a phenomenon in context and to reach an understanding of the social, historical, economic and political contexts from which it has emerged. Therefore, the whole phenomenon is under study and approached holistically as a complex system.

For qualitative researchers, the social world cannot be simplified without missing important factors that are not easily quantifiable. Using a holistic approach, qualitative researchers gather data on multiple aspects of a setting under study, in order to assemble a comprehensive and complete picture of the social dynamic, of a particular situation or programme under study. This differs from the logic and procedures of many quantitative approaches where 'independent' and 'dependent' variables are identified and isolated, and then statistically manipulated. The statistical findings are then used to draw inferences about relationships between these measured variables.

Types of qualitative methods

Qualitative methods can be divided into two types: human-to-human and 'artefactual' methods (Guba & Lincoln 1981, Lincoln 1992). Human-to-human methods include interviewing, participant and non-participant observation, and focus groups. Artefactual methods are those that include the use of documents such as letters, memoranda, reports and diaries. The following is a brief discussion of the different methods used in qualitative inquiry.

Interviews

Interviews are often used in health research to explore how users feel about services they are offered, or to understand attitudes and perceptions underlying certain health and illness behaviours. They are used to gain knowledge about how different people interpret and experience the world around them, allowing researchers to gain access to these views, and to explore and find out why they have emerged. In this situation the researcher is interactive and sensitive to the language and concepts used by an informant. They aim to explore what the informant says in order to uncover new areas or ideas often inaccessible by quantitative methods. For example, interviews can be useful for exploring patients' and carers' experiences of particular treatments. In a study by Davies et al (1996), semi-structured interviews were used to explore patients' and relatives' perspectives of the value of radiotherapy for malignant cerebral glioma. By using the semi-structured approach, the researchers were able to expand on specific issues, while allowing patients and relatives to speak about any matters that affected them. The interviews revealed that relatives were much more likely to be aware of poor prognosis than were patients themselves, who were generally unaware of it. This lack of awareness made it difficult to discuss the issue of satisfaction with some patients. Of the patients who were aware, while they made negative comments about the use of radiotherapy, they were generally not dissatisfied with it. The authors concluded that patients' perceptions of the value of radiotherapy were closely tied to the patients' understanding of their condition.

While the distinction is often made between interviews that are structured and those that are unstructured, it is generally accepted that it is impossible to carry out any interview without having some degree of structure. Therefore, qualitative interviews are distinguished by the degree to which they are standardised. Denzin (1970) identified three different types of interviews: standard schedules, non-schedule standardised and non-standardised interviews (Box 6.1).

Focus groups

A focus group is a group interview that uses the communication *between* informants to generate data (Kitzinger 1995). It is important to note that with focus group research, a researcher is interested in the interaction as well as what is actually said.

Focus groups can be useful when a researcher wants to explore something that may not be very clear in informants' minds. Focus groups can allow informants to express and clarify their views in ways that are not easily accomplished in one-to-one interviews. They are recommended for use with informants who feel that they have nothing to say or are deemed 'unresponsive'. By participating in a discussion, these particular informants may find it easier to uncover how they really feel about something.

Box 6.1   Three types of interview identified by Denzin (1970)

- *Standard schedule* The wording and order of all questions is exactly the same for each respondent. These are also referred to as 'structured' interviews and the research instrument is administered in the same way each time. The use of standardised questions raises issues about whether the research is truly qualitative. However, structured interviewing using open-ended questions does allow informants some flexibility in how they respond. Consequently it can fall (just!) within the domain of qualitative research.

- *Non-schedule standardised* The researcher begins with a list of pre-identified themes or information required, but the actual phrasing and order of the questioning is determined by the flow of the conversation. In this way, the research attempts to maintain a 'conversation-like' tone but also gain answers to very particular questions. For example, Litva (1997) wanted to explore lay perceptions of health, illness and disease. A list of pre-determined themes was used to ensure that all the informants were asked about the same issues.

- *Non-standardised interviews*   There is no specific set of questions or themes and questions are not asked in any particular order. Usually a researcher covers only one or two issues and questions asked are driven by what an informant says in the interview and consist mostly of probing for clarification (Britten 1995).

Using open-ended questions, the researcher allows the group to identify and pursue their own priorities using their own vocabulary. People use many forms of expression – sarcasm, joking, anecdotes, arguing – and focus groups enable the researcher to access these different forms of discourse. This method has been used to explore the experiences of different groups of people in relation to disease, treatment and use of health services. Because focus groups can be culturally sensitive, they are ideal for exploring the perceptions held by various ethnic groups. Farooqi et al (2000) used focus groups with randomly selected South Asians living in Leicester to explore their perceptions of the risks of lifestyle factors for coronary heart disease.

A range of views were uncovered that included varying levels of understanding of risk factors for coronary heart disease. For example, many of the informants perceived stress to be a major risk factor, and identified barriers to improving lifestyle, such as how to cook traditional Indian food more 'healthily'. The group also revealed that language difficulties were a barrier to accessing health services.

Focus groups can be useful for exploring attitudes and needs of health professionals, as well as exploring how clinical evidence is translated into practice. For example, Coenen et al (2000) used focus groups to explore general practitioners' diagnostic and therapeutic decisions regarding adult patients presenting with complaints of coughing. They found that decisions to prescribe antibiotics for coughing were often weighed against and influenced by the perceived effect that not prescribing treatment might have on the doctor–patient relationship. This led Coenen et al (2000) to conclude that clinical indicators play only one part in therapeutic decision-making.

Observational methods

Observational methods are used by qualitative researchers in order to develop a systematic, detailed observation of behaviour and talk, by watching and recording what people say (Mays & Pope 1995). The researcher enters the social world or contexts in which informants exist – as opposed to bringing them to another environment – and attempts to collect data systematically in an unobtrusive manner. In this way, observational methods are said to occur in a naturalistic setting. The goal of participant observation is to grasp the informant's 'point of view, their relation to life, to realise their vision of the world' (Malinowski 1922). The decision to use observational methods is influenced by the extent to which the activities and interactions of a setting are felt to give meaning to the phenomena being investigated (Bogdewic 1992).

Gold (1958) and Junker (1960) identify four different types of observational roles defined by the amount of participation by the researcher: participant, participant observer, observing participant and observer (Box 6.2).

The data obtained from observational methods are usually in the form of 'thick descriptions' of the people, contexts, conversa-

Box 6.2 Four types of observational role

■ *Participant* The researcher often hides their identity and attempts to become immersed in the day-to-day activities and the setting of the informants. There is often the danger of becoming too immersed in the community under investigation and losing one's critical standpoint. At this point the researcher begins to identify completely with the group being studied and completely loses their critical stance.

■ *Participant observer* The researcher overtly observes the informants and there is prolonged engagement with the informants but at the same time restricting involvement in the informants' daily activities. The researcher's critical stance is maintained but less so than for observing participation.

■ *Observing participant* This relationship is more formal than the previous one. The researcher is overt and known to the informants but there is usually no prolonged engagement and contact is likely to be briefer than for participating observers.

■ *Observer* This is similar to experimental designs. The researcher only observes and does not become involved in the informants' activities.

tions, sounds, and smells, in the form of detailed fieldnotes, often supplemented by audio/video recording or photographs.

Observational methods are particularly well suited for the study of organisations and how people within them perform their functions. They can uncover behaviours or routines of which informants themselves may be unaware. This method has been used to explore the role that clinical evidence plays in some surgical decision-making. Bloor (1976) observed at an ear, nose and throat outpatient clinic to uncover how decisions to admit children for tonsillectomy were made. By observing how surgeons made decisions to operate, Bloor found that clinical research evidence was not the only factor when making a decision to perform a tonsillectomy. While some surgeons would wait for clinical signs as the chief indicator for surgery, others would operate if there was evidence that tonsillitis was severely disrupting a child's daily activities, particularly school.

In order to understand the role of pharmaceutical consultation in patient health-seeking behaviour, Hassell et al (1997) combined participant observation with in-depth interviews to study advice-giving in community pharmacies. The authors found that patients use pharmacies as the first 'port of call' for many minor ailments, often preferring the pharmacist's advice to their GP's. The study findings highlighted the role that pharmacies play in keeping certain disorders from the doctor's surgery. They also demonstrated the potential value of closer partnerships between the community pharmacy and general practice.

Methods based on texts

Qualitative methods based on texts depend on the collection and analysis of different types of documents. The use of textual sources or documents has been a relatively neglected method in qualitative research (Atkinson & Coffey 1997). There are three categories of documents commonly used: informal, formal and visual (Box 6.3).

It may be difficult to understand the contribution that artefacts or document analysis can make to evidence-based medicine. However, in a study by Miller et al (1999), diaries were used to collect the illness experiences of patients suffering from lower back pain. The authors found that diaries elicited useful and diverse information about their illness experiences, supporting the relevance of a biopsychosocial approach to management of their condition. In addition, they concluded that there was some evidence of benefit to the patient from having written down and expressed their illness experiences.

Box 6.3 Three types of document used in qualitative research

- *Informal*: includes naturally occurring written accounts of everyday life such as unstructured diaries, autobiographical accounts and letters.
- *Formal*: includes documents constructed about everyday life such as death certificates, structured diaries, medical notes, various public records, timetables, or work rosters.
- *Visual*: documents with a visual quality such as photographs, advertisement, poster, film, map charts or video.

A well-known study by Bloor (1994) combined document analysis with interviews to explore the level of consistency in the death certification process. Drawing on a sample of doctors responsible for a higher than average number of death certificates, Bloor asked them to fill in a dummy death certificate, based upon a short summary which described the circumstances of death of a patient. Bloor asserts that it was the combination of interviews and document analysis that helped reveal the inconsistencies arising in what doctors listed as the cause of death, even when all were provided with the same information.

Many written or visual documents can form the basis for a textual analysis. For example, the personal account by Rier (2000) of being in an intensive care unit was based upon a notebook he used to communicate with others while he was intubated. This was complemented by faxes sent by his partner to his parents living overseas, his medical notes and, later on, speaking with nurses and people who had visited him. Inadvertently, these documents allowed him to reconstruct an experience usually unavailable to researchers, but also inaccessible to himself, as many of his memories about the event were lost. The result of Rier's work is a detailed and illuminating account of being a critically ill patient in an intensive care unit.

Appraising qualitative research

Within qualitative research there is a great deal of debate around the issue of the need for criteria to assess qualitative research. This debate is complicated by the diversity of opinion between qualitative researchers from different traditions as to the aims of qualitative research, and hence what constitutes good practice (Sandelowski 1986). While some feel that the search for standard criteria is misconceived (Smith 1984), the majority recognise the importance of establishing appropriate criteria to assess the quality of qualitative research proposals and findings generated from qualitative data (Denzin & Lincoln 1994, Hammersley 1990, Lincoln & Guba 1985, Murphy et al 1998). Although there is contention (Kirk & Miller 1986), it is well recognised that, as qualitative research emerges from a methodological paradigm distinct from quantitative research, a specific and relevant set of criteria needs to be developed (Lincoln & Guba 1985).

Within health research, there have been several attempts to develop checklists, guidelines or sets of criteria (Dingwall et al 1998, Mays & Pope 1995, Murphy et al 1998, Seale & Silverman 1997). Depending upon the author, particular criteria have received more or less emphasis than others. There is always a risk that the content of these sets of guidelines, criteria or checklists serves simply to discourage potential researchers from trying to conduct qualitative research (Chapple & Rogers 1998). Barbour (2000) recently stated that the uncritical adoption of different 'qualitative techniques' (such as triangulation, respondent checking, thick description) is likely to result in a case of the tail wagging the dog, and in itself does not create rigorous qualitative research.

It is important to recognise that the techniques we present are not exhaustive and that there is disagreement within the qualitative research community (see Smith 1984). There can be no algorithmic criteria produced that can unproblematically judge the quality of qualitative research (Hammersley 1992). Box 6.4 provides a simple overview of the criteria that are covered in the following section but we emphasise that it cannot be treated as a rigid checklist. Instead we present the criteria in the form of critical questions that should be considered when appraising a piece of qualitative research. Each criterion is explained before describing the techniques used to address it. It is common to find that the same technique is often used to satisfy two or more criteria (e.g. thick descriptions). There may be an inclination to turn this into a 'checklist' approach to assessing qualitative research. The assessment of qualitative research – indeed any research – requires judgement and a good understanding of the method and what it is trying to accomplish. In order to educate the readers' judgement, in the following section we propose that the quality of qualitative research is assessed based upon a critical assessment of how well the issues of credibility, transferability, dependability and confirmability are addressed.

Appraising credibility: Would those having the experience recognise the researchers' account of it?

In quantitative research, validity is the extent to which a proposition is generated, refined, tested and matches what occurs in human life. However, this concept rests upon the assumption

Box 6.4 How has the researcher used the following techniques to ensure the credibility, transferability, dependability and confirmability of the findings?

- *Credibility*
  Respondent/member checking
  Negative case analysis
  Triangulation (source/data, methods, investigator, theoretical)
  Constant comparative analysis
- *Transferability*
  Thick description
  Theoretical triangulation
- *Dependability*
  Flexibility in research design
  Mechanical recording devices
  Verbatim transcription
  Researcher triangulation
  Respondent/member checking
- *Confirmability*
  Thick description
  Reflexivity

that there is a single reality. Qualitative research embraces the notion of multiple, constructed realities. Therefore, it is difficult to develop a single benchmark against which the truth-value of its claims can be judged. Consequently, Lincoln & Guba (1985) and Hammersley (1990) suggest that validity in qualitative research should be assessed by the extent to which an account accurately and plausibly represents the social phenomena under scrutiny. Key to this is the question of how well a description of a phenomenon under study is recognised both by those who have experienced it and those outside the experience (Lincoln & Guba 1985). There are several techniques used in qualitative research to ensure this, and hence the validity of its findings. These are generally accepted as being member checking, negative case analysis, triangulation and constant comparison analysis.

Respondent or member checking

> Has the author used member checking? If so, do they explain how comments from informants were handled?

Member checking refers to the process of feeding back the researcher's interpretations of the data to informants to determine whether they can recognise and agree with them (Bloor 1983). It can also involve feeding back transcripts to informants to ask them to clarify or elucidate certain points. Lincoln & Guba (1985) assert that respondent checking is a powerful tool to check the credibility of the research findings because it allows the researcher to check and correct interpretations, gain additional information, and get the informants' seal of approval, thus confirming that the researcher 'got it right'.

Member checking, however, is not unproblematic (Bloor 1983, Emerson & Pollner 1988). There may be differences or tensions between how the researcher and the informant interpret the informant's world. Consequently, member checking may be limited to asking informants if the researcher's interpretation represents a *reasonable* interpretation of their accounts. There is also the question of how much researchers can reasonably ask of informants. Informants, having already allowed the researcher to explore their world, often do not want additional contact which will take up more of their time and energy. Informant checking also puts informants potentially in the position of being critical of the researcher, something they may not be prepared to do.

Despite these limitations, member checking, especially when combined with other strategies for ensuring the validity or credibility of qualitative research, is a useful strategy for increasing confidence in the validity of the findings. If member checking is used, the researcher should clearly indicate how they did it, as well as how comments were handled.

Negative case analysis

> Did the researcher actively seek out discomfirming or inconsistent evidence and report how it was dealt with?

There is a risk in qualitative data analysis of making the data look more 'ordered' or regular than it actually is. In order to prevent this, negative case analysis is used. Negative case analysis refers to the process of actively searching for cases that appear to be inconsistent with the emerging analysis (Glaser & Strauss 1965). By systematically seeking out exceptional cases, the researcher can refine their analysis (Silverman 1989) until they develop constructs that incorporate most of the available data. By demonstrating in their detailed account or audit trail how they sought out negative cases and how they dealt with them, the researcher therefore strengthens the credibility of research findings.

Triangulation

> Did the author attempt to search for negative cases or alternative explanations using either different methods or researchers or sources?
> Have they illustrated their findings using quotes from several different informants?
> Have they used more than one method for collecting data?
> During analysis, was more than one point of view used to develop coding structure and final accounts?
> Has the researcher attempted to apply multiple theoretical perspectives to interpret the data?

Triangulation is considered one of the most significant strategies for strengthening the credibility of qualitative research (Lincoln & Guba 1985, Miller & Crabtree 1994, Morse 1994). The underlying assumption of triangulation is that if multiple sources, methods, investigators or theories provide similar findings, their credibility is strengthened. Denzin (1970) identifies four different triangulation strategies:

- *Source/data triangulation*: refers to the use of more than one data source to develop an account. This commonly involves including different informants from the same setting and presenting quotes from several different informants to support a finding.
- *Method triangulation*: qualitative findings increase in validity when different and contrasting methods of collection produce

very similar results from the same sample set (Bloor 1997). It is not uncommon for findings produced from quantitative methods to be triangulated with qualitative findings but more commonly a phenomenon is approached using two or more of the qualitative methods outlined in the previous section.

■ *Investigator triangulation*: involves multiple investigators studying the same phenomena independently to see if they arrive at the same results. It is most commonly employed during data analysis but it is not uncommon to have two researchers collecting data. It can also involve exposing the data to more than one researcher so that alternative perspectives can be entertained and alternative interpretations explored.

■ *Theoretical triangulation*: refers to approaching the data with multiple perspectives and hypotheses in mind so that different theoretical points of view can be compared and contrasted.

Researchers use triangulation in many different ways. Methods and source triangulation are the most commonly used and theoretical triangulation tends to be the least common. The question is, of course, not simply whether triangulation has been used, but how well it has been used and whether in a meaningful manner.

Constant comparative analysis

> Did the author use the constant comparison method of analysis and was this clearly reported?

The constant comparative method means that the researcher is always seeking out cases in the dataset during data collection that support or 'shape' provisional hypothesis (Silverman 2000). This can be done while collecting data, but Glaser and Strauss (1967) assert that it can also involve inspecting and comparing all the different types of data after they have been collected. This can include quantitative data, observations, written accounts – all the different types of data that can arise in a single study. This usually requires a dataset that is fully transcribed. Using a small part of the dataset the researcher develops a set of categories or themes. These are tested out (and sometimes modified) as the researcher incorporates the remaining dataset. The goal of this strategy is to 'use' the entire dataset instead of just parts of it, in order to avoid the temptation to select only those bits of data that fit with the current analytic argument (ten Have 1998). In this way, the constant comparative method ensures that the dataset is given comprehensive treatment.

Appraising transferability: How well can the findings fit contexts outside the study situation?

Has the researcher provided a detailed account of the research context and informants?
Has the research produced a theoretical inference that can be examined in other settings?

The quantitative notion of generalisability refers to the extent to which findings from research produced in one setting are applicable to other similar settings. However, this perspective downplays or ignores the importance of time and context upon research findings. Within the qualitative paradigm, it is accepted that findings are highly contextualised, partial and temporal. Consequently, direct comparability between research settings is almost impossible. Qualitative researchers have opted for the concept of transferability instead of seeking to be able to generalise from their findings. In utilising the concept of transferability (Lincoln & Guba 1985) qualitative researchers recognise that, while direct comparisons between research settings cannot be made, some similarities will exist and it is possible to develop working hypotheses that can potentially transfer between different settings. Transferability requires providing sufficient descriptive detail for another researcher to be able to make an informed judgement about whether this is likely to be the case (Kennedy 1979). Being able to evaluate the possibility of transferability depends heavily upon the provision of a 'thick description' (Geertz 1973) or a very detailed account of the methodological and interpretive strategy in the form of field notes.

Thick description

Was the researcher explicit about every step of the research process?
This should include detailed descriptions of:

- Research context(s)
- Site selection and sampling strategy
- How informants were accessed
- How data were collected and recorded
- How analysis was conducted.

Transferability greatly depends on other researchers being able to determine how research findings are produced. This is achieved through the provision of 'thick descriptions'. These provide a thorough and detailed account of: the contexts or settings where the research took place; of sampling strategies; how informants or settings were accessed; and of the process of data collection and analysis. Also referred to as 'audit trails' by Guba & Lincoln (1989) and 'auditability' by Beck (1993), thick descriptions allow other researchers to examine the processes by which the researchers have arrived at their conclusions. Consequently, transferability is assessed by the extent to which the researchers have made transparent the decision trail that led them to their conclusions.

It must be noted that the provision of a thick description of the research process is often unseen in published qualitative research. When reading qualitative journal papers, it cannot be inferred that the lack of a detailed audit trail means that one was not done. In many cases, the authors of such papers have written a detailed account of their audit trail, often in the form of fieldnotes, which is available for exploration and inspection upon request.

Appraising dependability: Given the instability of the social world, how has the researcher been able to produced plausible accounts?

The quantitative notion of internal reliability refers to the extent to which, given a set of previously generated concepts, new researchers would match these concepts with the data in a similar way. Within qualitative research, this poses difficulty for a research paradigm committed to naturalistic inquiry, where the researcher is the research instrument (LeCompte & Goetz 1982) and the social world is constantly changing. Guba & Lincoln (1989) suggest that another way of approaching the issue of internal reliability is to determine how plausible or dependable the accounts produced are, *given* the instability of the social world. Therefore the concept of dependability refers to the degree to which it is possible to deal with instability/idiosyncrasy and design-induced change and produce plausible accounts (Kirk & Miller 1986).

As qualitative researchers do not believe that accepting the inevitability of changes in reality produces unreliable findings, the emphasis is upon design/researcher-induced changes. The techniques used in qualitative research to improve the dependability of the research include: flexible research design; use of mechanically recorded data; and verbatim transcription. Researcher triangulation and member checking are also used to ensure the dependability of the accounts.

Flexibility in research design

> Did the researcher encounter anything unexpected when entering the field?
> Did the researcher report how they adapted to any unexpected changes?

Given that the social world is constantly changing and often unpredictable, qualitative inquiry cannot be completely specified in advance of fieldwork. Whilst a study design will have an initial question and plans for exploring this question, the naturalistic and inductive nature of the inquiry makes it both impossible and inappropriate to specify operational variables, state hypotheses or finalise a research instrument or sampling strategy (Patton 1990). Consequently much of qualitative research design unfolds as the study progresses.

Due to the requirements of funding agencies or dissertation committees, qualitative researchers tend to develop a strategy for exploring a particular phenomenon before entering the field. When in the field, the researcher will need to demonstrate a high level of tolerance for ambiguity or uncertainty, and attempt to deal with it in a pragmatic and flexible manner. For example, if the researcher finds during the course of a study that their original ideas about how to gain access to informants is not working, they will need to re-evaluate their approach and decide upon a more appropriate strategy or strategies. The researcher is required to demonstrate what happened during fieldwork, why it happened, and how it might impact on the research findings in the thick description of data collection.

Use of mechanic recording devices and transcripts

> Has the researcher used mechanical recording devices?
> Did they obtain permission to use these devices from the informant(s)?
> How were the tapes handled?
> What rules were followed for transcription?
> How were any identifying features handled?

The dependability of qualitative research is closely related to the quality of the data (Silverman 1993). Using mechanical devices for recording data is a common strategy to ensure the quality and accuracy of qualitative data, thus increasing its dependability. Mechanical devices produce highly reliable accounts, as they are not dependent on the researcher's ability to recall what took place. Mechanical recordings are usually done with the use of a video camera or a tape recording machine. Researchers are required to report what type of device was used and if permission was given by the informant to use it. Researchers who do not gain the informant's permission prior to recording an interaction are considered to be ethically questionable.

Tapes are transcribed verbatim, often according to a specific set of rules (see Poland 1995), to create the raw materials that researchers work from. At this point in the process, identifying features are often removed in order to protect the anonymity of the informants. If anonymisation of the data has taken place, it is essential that it be reported. In addition, the researcher should explain how tapes were stored to protect the identities of informants.

The result of this process is a highly detailed and publicly accessible representation of the interactions under investigation. This allows other researchers to examine the data and assess its credibility and dependability.

Assessing confirmability: Has the study explained how the researcher might have affected the research findings?

The concept of confirmability focuses attention on both the investigator and interpretations. What is known by quantitative researchers as external reliability, poses many problems for qualitative researchers. External reliability refers to the extent to which independent researchers would discover the same phenomena or generate the same findings in the same or similar settings. This requires neutrality or objectivity on the part of the researcher. Confirmability is suggested as a qualitative parallel for the quantitative notion of external reliability. Confirmability refers to the degree to which findings are determined by the respondents and condition of the inquiry, and not by the biases of the inquirer (Lincoln & Guba 1985). Thus, qualitative researchers are expected to account for their interests and motivations by showing how they have affected the interpretations. One strategy, described previously, is to provide a thick description of how decisions were made during every stage of the research process. Another is the technique called reflexivity.

Reflexivity

> Has the researcher(s) attempted to be reflexive about their impact on the research process either in the form of an autobiographical account or in their analysis?

Within quantitative research, the goal is always to limit the influence of the researcher on the research findings through standardisation of procedures. However, in qualitative research, the commitment is to a naturalistic setting and this partly requires asking questions in a way that is appropriate to the person you are speaking with. There is also a recognition that in order to study the social world one must enter it (Hammersley & Atkinson 1995). While objectivity or distance is not possible, reflexivity allows for researchers to limit the impact they have on what is produced.

Reflexivity refers to sensitivity to the ways in which a researcher's presence affects data collection, or how their own assumptions have shaped the data analysis. This requires a certain degree of self-conscious reflection upon the way in which the research outputs have been shaped by the person who has conducted it. It requires being explicit, often in the form of an autobiographical account (see Litva 1997), about the personal and theoretical assumptions the researcher brings to the research. It also requires recognition of how such things as the researcher's social position, appearance, voice, age, gender and other characteristics will influence the research process (Silverman 1993). The use of the technique of reflexivity is most common in the analysis of data, where the author may reflect on how they have shaped or influenced what has been found.

It must be noted here that editorial limits on the length of journal papers means that authors cannot always provide a detailed account of how they addressed the issue of confirmability. Thus it may often appear to be poorly handled in qualitative papers.

How can qualitative research inform clinical practice?

Finally, we turn to the question of how qualitative research can inform clinical practice. Evidence-based medicine is the 'conscientious, explicit, and judicious use of current best evidence in making decisions about the care of individual patients' (Sackett et al 1996). It is now recognised that the *practice* of evidence-based medicine requires a strategy that combines the best available evidence with individual clinical expertise and patient preferences, in order to devise a strategy that is most appropriate for the patient (Muir Gray 1997). The advantage that qualitative methods bring to the practice of evidence-based medicine is that they can systematically examine the kinds of questions that cannot usually be answered by experimental methods (Green & Britten 1998). Some examples of questions that qualitative methods can address are presented in Box 6.5.

Qualitative methods can be used to explore the impact of patient attitudes and beliefs on their care. For example, clinical evidence indicates that giving thrombolytic therapy early in a heart attack episode maximises its benefit and prevents premature death and disability (Weston et al 1994). However Rushton et al (1998), in a qualitative study undertaken to explore reasons for delays in the delivery of thrombolytic therapy for patients having heart attacks, found that patients often delay seeking treatment because they fail to recognise their symptoms as cardiac in origin. As a result, the window of opportunity by which thrombolytic therapy can be given and have the best outcome is inadvertently reduced.

A qualitative study by Howitt & Armstrong (1999) demonstrates how patient attitudes to the risks and benefits of treatment can impact upon clinical decision-making. These authors explored uptake of anti-thrombotic treatment for atrial fibrillation. They

---

Box 6.5 Examples of clinical evidence questions that lend themselves to qualitative research methods

- Why do patients seek or delay medical care/treatment?
- Where else do patients seek help?
- What are the factors that facilitate or limit help-seeking behaviour?
- What are patients' perceptions of causes of their illnesses and how do these differ from those of health care professionals?
- What is the impact of the doctor–patient relationship upon treatment decisions?
- What concerns do health care professionals have about treatments?
- Why do health care professionals make particular decisions about patient management?
- What factors contribute to or inhibit patient adherence to treatment?
- What do patients perceive their treatment needs to be?
- What are the factors that inhibit or facilitate practitioners or health care teams in following particular clinical guidelines?

---

identified patients who were at increased risk of thromboembolism, and educated them on the relevance of aspirin and warfarin as preventative treatment. The study revealed that giving patients an active role in deciding whether to take warfarin tended to result in a low uptake. One of the conclusions of the study was that a barrier to the implementation of evidence-based medicine is that patients must consent to treatment. In deciding whether to give consent, patients draw on their own understandings of the risk of having a stroke against the costs of taking the treatment. Howitt & Armstrong (1999) suggest that while patients have most to benefit from the implementation of effective treatment, without their support evidence-based medicine is limited in its applicability.

Qualitative methods are also effective for providing in-depth contextualised accounts of the role of practitioners' attitudes and beliefs (see Tomlin et al 1999) for turning evidence into practice. For example Grol et al (1998) sought to uncover what factors influenced whether or not Dutch general practitioners followed clinical guidelines. Using an observational approach they found that practitioners' perceptions of particular attributes of clinical guidelines strongly influenced how well they were followed.

Another area of decision-making which qualitative methods can illuminate is the question as to why and when patients decide to seek professional care. A study using in-depth interviews with parents living in the southeast of England explored the process by which they decided whether or not to call the doctor out (Houston & Pickering 2000). The study findings showed that parents employed reasonable strategies – such as waiting to see if their child improved or using over-the-counter drugs such as paracetamol – when attempting to manage their child's illness. It was only when they began to become aware of their limitations and feared doing the wrong thing that parents thought about calling the doctor out. The authors of the study concluded by stating that health professionals needed to re-think the 'problem' of out-of-hours calls. Parents were struggling not so much with a lack of knowledge on how to treat minor illness as with the problems of coping with uncertainty.

The above examples are all studies where qualitative methods were used as a single strategy. In conjunction with quantitative methods, qualitative approaches may also be better at identifying the appropriate variables to be measured or questions to be asked. Insights from qualitative data can help to develop quantitative instruments that are more sensitive to respondents' meanings and interpretations (Coyle & Williams 2000). Black (1994) argues that qualitative methods are very proficient at providing explanations for anomalous or unexpected quantitative findings as well as generating hypotheses about areas that are not well understood.

It is because of their ability to answer questions which cannot be addressed by experimental methods that qualitative approaches have a place alongside randomised controlled trials and meta-analysis in producing applicable clinical evidence, thus contributing to the effective practice of evidence-based medicine. This will require qualitative research that explores questions relevant to practice (Barbour 2000).

Conclusions

In this chapter we have explored the value of qualitative methods for the practice of evidence-based medicine. We began the chapter by asserting that qualitative methods have a very active role to play in the development of applicable and appropriate approaches to health care research. There are many qualitative strategies that can be used to explore questions that are relevant to the practice of evidence-based medicine. When selecting which, careful thought must be put into what is the most appropriate strategy to answer the question being asked. Only when used appropriately can qualitative methods become a powerful research tool for addressing clinical practice questions.

It is essential that if qualitative research methods are to be used in the production of clinical evidence, they are used in a systematic and careful way to produce findings that are of the highest quality. In the latter part of this chapter, we define four criteria that can be used to assess the quality or 'goodness' of qualitative research and the techniques used to address each criterion. The application of qualitative methods into evidence-based medicine will undoubtedly engender some very challenging and exciting results. It will contribute not only to the production of clinically and cost-effective treatment, but also of clinical practice that is appropriate for everyone.

Summary

- The purpose of the qualitative approach is to produce insights on the social world that are developed within the contexts in which it exists. It focuses upon the meanings, experiences and practices of those who are being investigated. It is inductive research that seeks to understand social phenomena within their own context, incorporating many different perspectives in order to provide a holistic perspective.

- Qualitative data collection is driven by what is the most appropriate strategy to explore the social phenomena under investigation. It can involve the use of interviews, focus groups, observations or investigation of texts.

- Because of the many traditions within qualitative research, it is necessary to avoid a checklist approach to evaluating qualitative research. Instead, evaluation should be considered in terms of critically assessing how different techniques have been used to increase the credibility, transferability, dependability and confirmability of the research.

■ Qualitative research can inform clinical practice by being able to examine the kinds of question that cannot be answered using experimental methods alone. By combining qualitative methods with quantitative approaches, the ability to produce applicable clinical evidence is greatly increased.

References

Atkinson P, Coffey A 1997 Analysing documentary realities. In: Silverman D (ed.) Qualitative research: theory, methods, and practice. London: Sage

Barbour RS 2000 Checklists for improving rigour in qualitative research: a case of the tail wagging the dog? British Medical Journal 322: 1115–1117

Beck CT 1993 Qualitative research: the evaluation of its credibility, fittingness and auditability. Western Journal of Nursing Research 15: 263–266

Black N 1994 Why we need qualitative research. Journal of Epidemiology and Community Health 48: 425–426

Bloor M 1976 Bishop Berkeley and the adenotonsillectomy enigma: an exploration of the social construction of medical disposals. Sociology 10: 43–61

Bloor M 1983 Notes on member validation. In: Emerson RM (ed.) Contemporary field research: a collection of readings. Boston: Little

Bloor M 1994 On the conceptualization of routine medical decision-making: death certification as a habitual activity. In: Bloor M, Taraborrelli P (eds) Qualitative studies in health and medicine. Aldershot: Avebury

Bloor M 1997 Techniques of validation in qualitative research: a critical commentary. In: Miller G, Dingwall R (eds) Context and method in qualitative research. London: Sage

Bogdewic SP 1992 Participant observation. In: Crabtree BF, Miller WL (eds) Doing qualitative research. London: Sage

Britten N 1995 Qualitative interviews in medical research. British Medical Journal 311: 251–253

Bryman A 1988 Quantity and quality in social research. London: Unwin Hyman

Chapple A, Rogers A 1998 Explicit guidelines for qualitative research: a step in the right direction, a defence of the 'soft' option or a form of sociological imperialism? Family Practice 15: 556–561

Coenen S, Van Royen P, Vermeire E, Hermann I, Denekens J 2000 Antibiotics for coughing in general practice: a qualitative decision analysis. Family Practice 17 (5): 380–385

Coyle J, Williams B 2000 An exploration of the epistemological intricacies of using qualitative data to develop a quantitative measure for user views of health care. Journal of Advanced Nursing 31(5): 1235–1243

Davies E, Clarke C, Hopkins A 1996 Malignant cerebral glioma – II: Perspectives of patients and relatives on the value of radiotherapy. British Medical Journal 313: 1512–1516

Denzin N 1970 The research act, 1st edn. Englewood Cliffs, NJ: Prentice Hall

Denzin N, Lincoln Y 1994 Entering the field of qualitative research. In: Denzin N and Lincoln Y (eds) Handbook of qualitative research. Thousand Oaks, CA: Sage

Dingwall R, Murphy E, Watson P, Greatbach D, Parker S 1998 Catching goldfish: quality in qualitative research. Journal of Health Services Research and Policy 3(3): 167–172

Emerson RM, Pollner M 1988 On members' responses to researchers' accounts. Human Organisation 47: 189–198

Farooqi A, Nagra D, Edgar T, Khunti K 2000 Attitudes to lifestyle risk factors for coronary heart disease amongst South Asians in Leicester: a focus group study. Family Practice 17(4): 293–297

Geertz C 1973 The interpretation of culture. New York: Basic Books.

Glaser BG, Strauss A 1965 The discovery of substantive theory: a basic strategy underlying qualitative research. American Behavioural Scientist 8: 5–12

Glaser BG, Strauss A 1967 The discovery of grounded theory. Chicago: Aldine

Gold RL 1958 Roles in sociological field observations. Social Forces 36: 217–223

Green J, Britten N 1998 Qualitative research and evidence based medicine. British Medical Journal 316: 1230–1232

Grol R, Dalhuijsen J, Thomas S, in t'Veld C, Rutten G, Mokkink H 1998 Attributes of clinical guidelines that influence use of guidelines in general practice: observational study. British Medical Journal 317: 858–861

Guba EG 1981 Criteria for assessing the trustworthiness of naturalistic inquiries. Educational Communication and Technology Journal 29: 75–92

Guba EG, Lincoln Y 1981 Effective evaluation. San Francisco: Jossey-Bass

Guba EG, Lincoln Y 1989 Fourth generation evaluation. Newbury Park, CA: Sage

Hammersley M 1990 Reading ethnographic research. New York: Longman

Hammersley M 1992 What is wrong with ethnography? London: Routledge

Hammersley M, Atkinson P 1995 Ethnography: principles in practice. London: Routledge

Hassell K, Noyce PR, Rogers A, Harris J, Wilkinson J 1997 A pathway to the GP: the pharmaceutical 'consultation' as a first port of call in primary care. Family Practice 14(6): 498–502

Houston AM, Pickering AJ 2000 'Do I don't I call the doctor': a qualitative study of parental perceptions of calling the GP out-of-hours. Health Expectations 3: 234–242

Howitt A, Armstrong D 1999 Implementing evidence based medicine in general practice: audit and qualitative study of antithrombotic treatment for atrial fibrillation. British Medical Journal 318: 1324–1327

Junker BH 1960 Field work: an introduction to the social science. Chicago: University of Chicago Press

Kennedy M 1979 Generalising from single case studies. Evaluation Quarterly 3: 661–678

Kirk J, Miller M 1986 Reliability and validity in qualitative research. Newbury Park, CA: Sage

Kitzinger J 1995 Introducing focus groups. British Medical Journal 311: 299–302

LeCompte M, Goetz JP 1982 Problems of reliability and validity in ethnographic research. Reviews of Educational Research 52: 31–60

Lincoln Y 1992 Sympathetic connections between qualitative methods and health research. Qualitative Health Research 2(4): 375–391

Lincoln Y, Guba EG 1985 Naturalistic inquiry. Newbury Park, CA: Sage

Litva A 1997 'Placing' lay perceptions of health and illness. PhD dissertation, McMaster University, Canada

Malinowski B 1922 Argonauts of the Western Pacific. London: George Routledge

Marshall C, Rossman G 1989 Designing qualitative research. London: Sage

Mays N, Pope C 1995 Observational methods in health care settings. British Medical Journal 311: 182–184

Miller BF, Crabtree B 1994 Clinical research. In: Denzin N, Lincoln Y (eds) Handbook of qualitative research. Thousand Oaks, CA: Sage

Miller J, Pinnington MA, Stanley IM 1999 The early stages of low back pain: a pilot study of patient diaries as a source of data. Family Practice 16(4): 395–401

Morse J 1994 Designing funded qualitative research. In: Denzin N, Lincoln Y (eds) Handbook of qualitative research. Thousand Oaks, CA: Sage

Muir Gray JA 1997 Evidence based health care: how to make health policy and management decisions. New York: Churchill Livingstone

Murphy E, Dingwall R, Greatbach D, Parker S, Watson P 1998 Qualitative research methods in health technology assessment: a review of the literature. Health Technology Assessment Report 2(16)

Patton MQ 1990 Qualitative evaluation and research methods. London: Sage

Poland B 1995 Transcription quality as an aspect of rigor in qualitative research. Qualitative Inquiry 1(3): 290–310

Popay J, Williams G 1998 Qualitative research and evidence-based health care. Journal of Royal Society of Medicine 91(35): 32–37

Pope C, Mays N 1995 Reaching the parts other methods cannot reach: an introduction to qualitative methods in health and health services research. British Medical Journal 311: 42–45

Rier DA 2000 The missing voice of the critically ill: a medical sociologist's first-person account. Sociology of Health & Illness 22(1): 68–93

Rushton A, Claton J, Calnan M 1998 Patients' action during their cardiac event: qualitative study exploring differences and modifiable factors. British Medical Journal 316: 1060–1065

Sackett DL, Rosenberg WMC, Muir Gray JA, Haynes RB, Richardson WS 1996 Evidence-based medicine: what it is and what it isn't. British Medical Journal 312: 71–72

Sandelowski M 1986 The problem of rigor in qualitative research. Annals of Advances in Nursing Science 8: 27–37

Seale CG, Silverman D 1997 Ensuring rigour in qualitative research. European Journal of Public Health 7: 379–384

Silverman D 1989 Telling convincing stories: a plea for a cautious positivism in case studies. In: Glassner B, Moreno JD (eds) The qualitative-quantitative distinction in the social sciences. Dordrecht: Kluwer Academic

Silverman D 1993 Interpreting qualitative data: methods for analysing talk, text and interaction. London: Sage

Silverman D 2000 Doing qualitative research: a practical handbook. London: Sage

Smith J 1984 The problem of criteria for judging interpretive inquiry. Educational Evaluation and Policy Analysis 6: 379–391

ten Have P 1998 Doing conversation analysis: a practical guide. London: Sage

Tomlin A, Huphrey C, Rogers S 1999 General practitioners' perceptions of effective health care. British Medical Journal 318: 1532–1535

Weston CFM, Penny WJ, Julian DG 1994 Guidelines for the early management of patients with myocardial infarction. British Medical Journal 308: 767–777

Further reading

Bloor M 1997 Techniques of validation in qualitative research: a critical commentary. In: Miller G, Dingwall R (eds.) Context and method in qualitative research. London: Sage

Denzin N, Lincoln Y (eds) 1994 Handbook of qualitative research. Thousand Oaks, CA: Sage

Hammersley M 1990 Reading ethnographic research. New York: Longman

Kirk J, Miller M 1986 Reliability and validity in qualitative research. Newbury Park, CA: Sage

Patton MQ 1990 Qualitative evaluation and research methods. London: Sage

7

Systematic reviews: what are they and how can they be used?

Rosalind L Smyth

Key points

- Systematic reviews use rigorous methods to reduce bias and can provide reliable summaries of relevant research evidence.
- Because systematic reviews include a comprehensive search strategy, appraisal and synthesis of research evidence, they can be used as shortcuts in the evidence-based process.
- The Cochrane Library, which is updated every 3 months, electronically, includes a database of up-to-date systematic reviews across the whole of health care.
- Critical appraisal of systematic reviews is necessary to ensure that they have been conducted to rigorous standards.
- Meta-analysis is a statistical technique used in systematic reviews. It can answer the questions 'does this intervention have a beneficial effect?' and if so, 'what is the size of that effect?'.

What are systematic reviews?

Reviews for health care professionals take many shapes and forms, depending on the type and expertise of the audience to which they are addressed. They may include chapters in textbooks, reports to expert committees and 'state of the art' reviews for clinical journals. The main purpose of these reviews is to bring their audience rapidly up to speed with the current information in specific clinical areas.

It is partly because of the explosion in information technology that we have come to rely increasingly on reviews. Indeed, evidence-based health care has been described as having 'the potential to rescue us from sinking in a sea of papers' (Bradley & Field 1995). It is because health professionals are bombarded by so many publications that may be relevant to their area of clinical practice on a weekly or monthly basis and it is impossible to sift through all of these, that they have come to rely on summaries of the evidence in the form of reviews. Many of these review articles are well researched, beautifully illustrated and highly entertaining and informative. However, as 'bottom line' summaries of what treatments, diagnostic tests, etc., are effective they may be misleading. One reason for this is that reviews are often written by acknowledged experts, who are likely to have already formed an opinion about what works, and who may not review the evidence in an unbiased manner. Another reason is that writing reviews is not always regarded as the most important academic activity and less time is devoted to it, than, for example, writing up original scientific research. So those writing the reviews may cut corners and rehash something they have written previously, rather than undertaking an exhaustive search and critical appraisal of all the evidence.

Let us take the example quoted by Professor Paul Knipschild in the book *Systematic Reviews* (Knipschild 1995). He describes how the distinguished biochemist Linus Pauling, writing in his book *How to Live Long and Feel Better* (Pauling 1986) quoted more than 30 trials that supported his contention that vitamin C could prevent the common cold. Knipschild and colleagues then went on to do their own 'systematic review' which showed that even large doses of vitamin C cannot prevent a cold although they may slightly decrease the duration and severity of a cold. A critical review of what Pauling had written showed that he had omitted a number of important studies which did not support the contention that he so enthusiastically proposed. There are now many examples that have shown that unsystematic or narrative reviews do not routinely incorporate all relevant up to-date scientific evidence.

This shortcoming has led to the notion that reviews need to be performed systematically. This means that the same rigours which we expect of people undertaking primary research should be demanded of reviewers undertaking this very important task of 'research synthesis' or 'secondary research'. You will have seen from Chapters 4 and 5 that in studies such as randomised controlled trials and diagnostic tests, the study can be designed so that bias is reduced or eliminated. Strategies such as blinding (or masking) investigators and participants in clinical trials to whether they are in the experimental or the control group may be introduced to prevent the human element of bias.

In the same way, strategies can be introduced to the reviewing process to eliminate the human element of bias caused, for example, by the reviewer having a strong opinion about whether the treatment under review works. The methodology of a systematic review is outlined in Box 7.1. The research needs to start with a protocol which first of all states clearly the hypothesis or question which the investigator is addressing. In Chapter 2 we have already discussed the importance of formulating an appropriate question. A systematic reviewer needs to define their question very precisely as everything else in the methodology will flow from this.

The search itself should be comprehensive, including not only electronic databases (e.g. MEDLINE) but also, where possible, accessing unpublished studies. This may seem odd, but there is a phenomenon known as 'publication bias'. For any intervention,

---

Box 7.1 How to conduct a systematic review

1. State objectives and hypotheses.
2. Outline eligibility criteria, stating types of study, types of participants, types of interventions and outcomes to be examined.
3. Perform a comprehensive search of all relevant sources for potentially eligible studies.
4. Examine the studies to decide eligibility (if possible with two independent reviewers).
5. Construct a table describing the characteristics of the included studies.
6. Assess methodological quality of included studies (if possible with two independent) reviewers.
7. Extract data (with a second investigator if possible) with involvement of investigators if necessary.
8. Analyse results of included studies, using statistical synthesis of data (meta-analysis), if appropriate.
9. Prepare a report of review, stating aims, materials and methods and describing results and conclusions.

there may be studies which do not show a clear benefit of the intervention compared with the control group and the evidence indicates that these are less likely to be published (Easterbrook et al 1991). By excluding unpublished studies from systematic reviews, this may bias the results of the review towards studies in which a benefit of the intervention was observed. Unpublished studies can be retrieved in a number of ways, none of which is perfect. One way of doing this is to search for abstracts of studies presented at conferences. These are available in the abstract books of relevant international conferences. Another common feature of systematic reviews, which may impair their quality, is that they may exclude study reports which are not published in English. Important information may be contained in such studies. For example, in the field of complementary medicine, many studies of acupuncture are published in non-English language journals, particularly those from China (Linde et al 2001).

The next step in the review is to decide what studies should be included. This should be done according to rigorous inclusion and exclusion criteria so that systematic bias can be avoided. These criteria should be stated in the review. The studies should be defined according to their design, the types of participants, the types of interventions and types of outcomes. For example, Poustie et al (2001) have published a review on the Cochrane Library entitled 'Oral protein calorie supplementation for children with chronic disease'. The review states that the types of participants were children aged 1–16 years with any defined chronic disease. Trials undertaken in children suffering from malnutrition who did not have an associated disease were not included.

The clear description of eligibility criteria can then be applied to all the studies retrieved from the search. Again, to reduce bias it is best if more than one reviewer can do this, working on their own. Two reviewers can then compare which studies they have independently included. They should have previously worked out a mechanism for deciding what to do if there are differences between their lists of included studies. This may mean involving a third reviewer. In the review of oral protein calorie supplementation, the search identified a very large number of studies conducted in children suffering from the effects of famine. The question of whether this intervention is effective in children with severe undernutrition in this setting is a very important one, but was not the question addressed in Poustie and colleagues' review and thus these studies were excluded.

Having decided which studies are eligible for inclusion, the reviewers need to tabulate their characteristics. This description should include the study methods, details of the participants, the precise nature of the interventions and the outcomes measured. You will notice that, in tabulating the study characteristics, the reviewers are describing the studies under the headings by which they have determined whether or not the study is eligible for inclusion in the review. For this reason, it may be helpful if steps 4 and 5 (Box 7.1) are done together. When reviewers are trying to determine whether a study is eligible for inclusion in a review, in many cases it is very obvious whether this is the case or not. However, by tabulating the characteristics of all studies where one or more reviewers thinks the study may be included, it will soon become apparent whether the inclusion criteria have been fulfilled. The final table of included studies, which all reviewers have agreed, will appear in the review and the readers can judge if the reviewers got it right. For each study excluded, the reviewers need to state, in the review, the reason for this exclusion, and again the reader can judge whether this is valid.

For example, Table 7.1 provides details of a study by Kalnins et al (1996) which was included in the review of oral protein calorie supplementation. This study included children and adults with cystic fibrosis over the age of 10, but the review addressed children only. However, the reviewers were able to obtain summary data on the children included in the trial by contacting the investigators in the original study. All the outcomes evaluated in the trial are listed and those which are evaluated in the review are asterisked. When reading a review, examination of the 'Characteristics of included studies' can help the reader to decide whether the review is applicable to their question. The reader may have in mind a particular age of patient or a specific type of intervention. If none of the studies have included this age of patient or type of intervention, then it is less likely that the review will be relevant.

The protocol should describe how the quality of the included studies will be assessed and how the data will be extracted and analysed. Again, it is best if these steps are performed by more than one person. The quality of the studies should be assessed using a checklist or scoring system. There are many of these now

Table 7.1 **Characteristics of included study**

Study	Methods	Participants	Interventions	Outcomes
Kalnins et al 1996	Quasi-randomised, parallel design	Cystic fibrosis patients aged > 10 years, < 90% ideal weight for height, or greater than 5% reduction in ideal weight for height over previous 3 months	High-calorie drinks to increase energy intake by 20% of predicted energy needs. Control group received nutritional counselling to increase energy intake by 20% of predicted energy needs by normal diet. Study period: 3 months	Z scores for weight and height;[a] percentage ideal weight for height;[a] anthropometric measures;[a] pulmonary function;[a] energy and nutrient intake;[a] faecal balance studies

[a]Protocol-defined outcome measures.
Data from Kalnins et al (1996).

available for the assessment of randomised controlled trials and other tools are being developed for other study designs. Generally, studies are graded according to whether they are of high, medium or low quality. It may be possible to separately analyse the high-quality studies. If the results of this analysis are the same as those obtained when studies of all standards of quality are analysed, this would reassure the reader that the results had not been biased by including low-quality studies. This is known as a 'sensitivity analysis'. In Knipschild's systematic review of vitamin C and the common cold, he identified 61 trials (Knipschild 1995). By applying a rigorous quality scoring, he found that only 15 were of high quality. When the trials which Knipschild included in his review were compared to the ones which Pauling considered, five of Knipschild's top 15 trials were not included by Pauling. Pauling did mention two preventative trials, which did not show any effect of vitamin C, but said that they were 'flawed'. Methodological quality of included studies is very important in a review, but it needs to be judged in an unbiased way.

The next steps in the review process are to extract the data and analyse them. When the reviewers stated their outcomes, they would have provided some indication of what measures they expected to find. The measures used in individual studies will be further described in the Table of study characteristics. For example, in Table 7.1 it will be seen that in the trial by Kalnins et al (1996) there were various measures of nutritional status, pulmonary function and energy intake. In extracting the data, the reviewers need to examine exactly what these measures are, for each trial, for the outcomes in which they are interested. They should draw up their own data extraction form, listing the measures made in each trial. In some situations statistical analysis of the results may not be possible. For example, slightly different measurements of outcomes may have been made in each of the included trials, and because of this they cannot be combined as one summary outcome measure. In this situation, reviewers should summarise the results of the individual studies, in narrative or tabular form, in the review. If a meta-analysis has not been possible, the results of the review (which should be the best possible summary of the evidence) are still robust.

Meta-analysis will be explained in detail later in this chapter. Essentially, in the analysis, sensible comparisons should be made and the results should be expressed in a way that is easy to understand. It is an often stated truism that 'no evidence of effect' is not the same as 'evidence of no effect' (Altman & Bland 1995). A review may conclude that there is no evidence to show that a treatment works, but this does not mean that the treatment does not work. Results from analysis of specific groups of patients (known as 'subgroups') should be interpreted with caution. The conclusions should be supported by the results and extravagant claims avoided.

By writing a protocol before they start the review, the reviewers are ensuring that their methods will not be influenced by prior knowledge of the studies that they are going to encounter. The methodology is made clear and if there are any potential sources of bias it is available for people to examine externally. It is this methodology that largely distinguishes a systematic review from a narrative or literature review.

Cochrane Systematic Reviews

In most descriptions of evidence-based practice a four-step approach is proposed (Box 7.2). It will be apparent from the previous discus-

> ### Box 7.2 Four steps in an evidence-based approach
>
> 1. Ask a clinically relevant question
> 2. Search for the best available external evidence
> 3. Critically appraise that evidence for its validity and relevance
> 4. Apply the evidence in clinical practice

sion that if you are able to directly access a systematic review which addresses the question posed, the systematic review would have already performed steps 2 and 3. Systematic reviews are therefore a 'shortcut' which the evidence-based practitioner can use to answer specific questions relating to clinical management. The very laborious task of searching and critical appraisal will already have been done by the reviewer. However, to be confident of this process one would need to be reassured that the systematic reviews being accessed were of high quality. In the end, rather than accessing databases of primary research studies such CINAHL or MEDLINE, would it not be much more convenient to access the database of systematic reviews? This is, in effect, what the Cochrane Database of Systematic Reviews, which is contained in the Cochrane Library, provides. The Cochrane Library has been referred to previously but here I shall discuss its merits as a source of systematic reviews.

There are two main problems with systematic reviews published in paper journals. The first is that in reviewing the evidence one wishes to be assured that the systematic review is up to date. In a paper journal, a systematic review can only be current up to the date of publication. This means that studies published subsequently will not have been included and these may change the Results and Conclusions of the systematic review. Secondly, systematic reviews require a lot of work, particularly in the meticulous searching for appropriate studies and their critical appraisal. It would be very disheartening indeed to discover just before you were due to submit a manuscript of a systematic review for publication that you had been 'pipped to the post' by somebody doing the same systematic review.

Both of these problems have been addressed by the Cochrane Collaboration. This is an international body of researchers who have responded to the challenge of the British epidemiologist Archie Cochrane. It was he who observed that 'it is surely a great criticism of our profession that we have not organised a critical summary by specialty or sub-specialty adapted periodically of all relevant randomised controlled trials' (Cochrane 1979). Systematic reviews published on the Cochrane Library are regularly updated. Later in the chapter, two systematic reviews from the Cochrane Library are used as examples. The version that has been used is Disk Issue 3, 2001. As you may be reading this some time later, these reviews are likely to have been updated and may contain new information. Duplication of effort is avoided as individual review groups within the Collaboration publish the titles of all systematic reviews as soon as the review process has started. The other important advantage of Cochrane Systematic Reviews is that they are of high quality. For example, Jadad et al (2000) have published an evaluation of reviews and meta-analyses of treatments used in asthma. Of the 50 reviews they included, 40 were found to have serious or extensive methodological flaws. They found that Cochrane Reviews had higher overall quality scores than those published in peer review journals.

The methodology for Cochrane Reviews has been developed by the Cochrane Collaboration and follows the same steps outlined in Box 7.1. Before the review is published, the protocol of the review is published first of all on the Cochrane Library so that readers of the library can examine the methodology before the results of the review are available. The coverage of the Cochrane Library does not extend to the whole of health care as yet. However, Disk Issue 3 2001 contained 1147 completed systematic reviews. I searched the Cochrane Library using the free text term nurs* and achieved hits on 328 of these 1147 reviews, so many of them are relevant to nursing practice. Clearly if one is able to identify a systematic review on the Cochrane Library that addresses the question of interest, this is a much quicker process than starting with other electronic databases. One can also be confident that all the relevant clinical studies will have been included.

Critical appraisal of systematic reviews

Box 7.3 shows a checklist adapted from Oxman (1994) for assessment of review articles. This checklist should clearly enable the reader to distinguish between narrative and systematic reviews, but should also enable the reader to assess the quality of system-

> **Box 7.3 Checklist for appraising systematic reviews**
>
> 1. Was the purpose of the review clearly stated?
> 2. Did the reviewers report a systematic and comprehensive search strategy to identify relevant studies?
> 3. Were inclusion and exclusion criteria for studies reported and were they appropriate (i.e. was selection bias avoided)?
> 4. Was the quality of included studies assessed appropriately?
> 5. Were the results of the included studies combined systematically and appropriately?
> 6. Were the conclusions supported by the data?

atic reviews and the rigour of the methodology. The latter point is particularly important as there is now evidence of considerable variation in quality of systematic reviews. The term 'systematic review' may have been applied to something inferior, in order to give it legitimacy.

Bias may be introduced as a result of the affiliations of the authors of the review. For example, a recent study by Barnes & Bero (1998) evaluated the quality of review articles on the health effects of passive smoking. They found that in these reviews a conclusion that passive smoking was not harmful was associated with authors who were affiliated with the tobacco industry. In Jadad's review of reviews on asthma (Jadad et al (2000)), all six reviews funded by the pharmaceutical industry were among the 40/50 with serious or extensive methodological flaws. All but one of these six studies had results and conclusions that favoured the intervention related to the companies sponsoring the review. These and other studies should make us aware that the heading 'systematic review' is not a guarantee that the results are reliable.

Understanding meta-analysis

Like all quantitative studies, systematic reviews often include a statistical analysis. This involves combining the data from the included studies in a process referred to as 'meta-analysis'. This analysis may be very powerful. The individual studies that make up a review are often small and unable, on their own, to detect whether or not a treatment is effective, but when the data from a number of similar small studies are combined, valid conclusions may be drawn. Often the terms 'meta-analysis' and 'systematic review' are used interchangeably. This is inappropriate because, as can be seen from Box 7.1, meta-analysis is simply one of the final steps in what must be a rigorous process. Statistical aggregation of the data in a meta-analysis does not mean that the individual studies included in a meta-analysis were reviewed systematically or appropriately. The most important part of the process is the one that I have already described, which refers to all the elements in the review process set up to prevent bias.

The Cochrane logo (Figure 7.1) is a stylised diagram of a meta-analysis from a systematic review. This systematic review included data from seven randomised controlled trials, which investigated the effect of corticosteroids administered to pregnant women who were about to deliver prematurely. The outcome examined was the survival of their infant. The vertical line is where these results would be expected to cluster if this treatment had a similar effect to the control group (placebo or no treatment) and each horizontal line represents the results of one trial. The shorter the line, the more certain the result, because the 95% confidence intervals are narrow. If the horizontal line lies entirely to the left of the vertical line the treatment has shown significant benefit. If it touches or crosses the vertical line then clear benefit was not demonstrated in that trial. If the horizontal line were to lie entirely to the right of the vertical line, then more babies

Figure 7.1 **The Cochrane Library logo indicating a meta-analysis of seven randomised controlled trials comparing corticosteroids versus no corticosteroids in pregnant women about to deliver prematurely. (From the Cochrane Library, Issue 3, 2001. Oxford: Update Software, with permission.)**

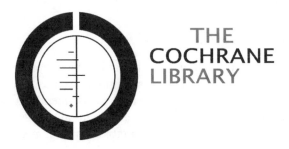

would have died in the treatment group than in the control group, i.e. the treatment would have been harmful. The trial at the top of the diagram was performed in 1972 and did show benefit, but the four subsequent trials did not. The sixth trial did show benefit and the seventh did not. On a simple 'vote count' (five of the trials showed no benefit) one might be persuaded not to use this intervention. However, when a systematic review was performed with meta-analysis and first reported in 1989 (Crowley 2001), this showed that corticosteroids administered to pregnant women reduced the odds of their babies dying by between 30% and 50%. This meta-analysis is indicated by the solid diamond at the bottom of the diagram.

Meta-analysis can answer two main questions about a treatment: 'Does this intervention have a beneficial (or harmful) effect?' and if so 'What is the size of that effect?' I will consider this with reference to specific examples. First, there are some terms used in expressing results that need to be explained. The first is known as the relative risk. The risk (or proportion, probability or rate) is the ratio of people with an event in a group compared with the total in that group. In Table 7.2, the risk of the outcome being present in group 1 is:

$$\frac{a}{a + c}$$

In 1992, a clinical trial published by Northeast et al (1990) compared two types of bandaging for the treatment of venous ulcers. One was of the use of elastic, high-compression bandaging, which is widely used in the UK, and the other was low-compression bandaging, used in standard practice in mainland Europe and Australia. The outcome that we will consider is complete healing of the ulcer within the trial period. There were 49 patients in the high-compression bandaging group and 52 in the low-compression group. Table 7.3 shows the numbers in each group which had complete healing. So the risk of complete ulcer healing in the

Table 7.2 A 2 × 2 table showing how results of a prospective study are represented

		Group 1	Group 2	Total
Outcome present	Yes	a	b	a + b
	No	c	d	c + d
	Total	a + c	b + d	n

Table 7.3 **Relation between complete ulcer healing and high-compression or low-compression bandaging**

		High compression	Low compression	Total
Complete healing	Yes	31	26	57
	No	18	26	44
	Total	49	52	101

Data from Northeast et al 1990.

high-compression group is 31/49 and the risk of complete healing in the low-pressure group is 26/52.

In a clinical trial the relative risk is the ratio of the risk in the intervention group to the risk in the control group. For this trial, the relative risk is:

$$\frac{31/49}{26/52} = \frac{0.63}{0.5} = 1.26$$

If the risk in the treatment group is the same as that in the comparison group the ratio will be 1. This means that there is no difference between the treatment and the comparison group.

The odds ratio is the ratio of the odds of an event in the treatment group compared to the odds of an event in the comparison group. The odds are the ratio of the number of people in a group with an event compared to the number without an event. So, looking again at Table 7.2, the odds of a patient in group 1 having the outcome present is:

$$a/c$$

In the Northeast trial, the odds of complete ulcer healing in the high-compression group is

$$31/18 = 1.72$$

In the low-compression group, the odds of complete ulcer healing is:

$$26/26 = 1.0$$

The odds ratio of complete ulcer healing in the two groups is:

$$1.72/1 = 1.72$$

If the odds of the event in the treatment group is the same as that in the comparison group then the odds ratio is again 1. That is, there is no difference between the treatment and comparison group.

Where the outcome of interest is rare, in Table 7.2, a will be very small and a/(a + c) will be approximately equal to a/c. Similarly b/(b + d) will approximately equal b/d. Thus, when the outcome is rare, the risks of the outcomes in the two groups will be very similar to the odds of the outcomes in the two groups and the relative risks will be very similar to the odds ratios.

Ninety-five per cent confidence intervals are an expression of how precise the estimate of the odds ratio or relative risk is. This gives an estimate of the range to 95% certainty that the true result for odds ratio or relative risk lies within the range stated.

Let us consider now a systematic review by Cullum et al (2001), which assessed the effectiveness of compression bandaging and stockings in treatment of venous leg ulcers. Included in this review was the comparison between high-compression and low-compression bandaging, which we have referred to previously. Three trials that made this comparison were found, including the study by Northeast et al (1990) described previously. This meta-analysis is illustrated in Table 7.4. The ratios shown in the column labelled 'Expt' indicate the number of patients in experimental group (elastic high compression) with complete healing compared with the

Table 7.4 Compression for venous leg ulcers. The comparison shown is for elastic high-compression versus inelastic compression (multilayer) (RR and 95% confidence interval). The outcome is complete healing in trial period (varying lengths)

Study	Expt n/N	Ctrl n/N	Peto OR (95%CI Fixed)	Weight %	Peto OR (95%CI Fixed)
Cullum	35/65	19/67	■	47.7	2.85 [1.43,5.68]
Gould	11/20	7/20	■	15.1	2.20 [0.64,7.52]
Northeast	31/49	26/52	■	37.2	1.71 [0.78,3.73]
Total (95%CI) Chi-square 0.93 (df = 2) Z = 3.35	77/134	52/139	◆	100.0	2.26 [1.40,3.65]

.10 .20   1   5   10
Inelastic better   Elastic better

Data from Cullum et al (2001).

total number of patients in that group. These risks are shown both for each individual study and, at the bottom, for the three studies combined. The term 'risk', as used here, is misleading, because the effect of ulcer healing is beneficial, but I have retained it for consistency. The total risk of healing in the high-compression bandage group is 77/134 (0.57), compared with the total risk of healing in the low-compression bandage group of 52/139 (0.37). The relative risk is the increased risk (or relative benefit) of complete healing in the high-compression bandage group compared with the low-compression bandage group, and is obtained by dividing the proportion of patients with complete healing in the high-compression bandage group by the proportion of patients with complete healing in the low-compression bandage group by the total, which is:

$$0.57/0.37 = 1.54$$

This represents the relative benefit increase for healing for the high-compression bandaging. You will recall that if the two treatments were equally effective this ratio should be 1.0. Because instead it is 1.54, this means there is a 54% relative benefit increase for healing in the high-compression bandaging group. Cullum et al (2001) calculated the 95% confidence intervals for the relative risks. For this relative benefit increase of 54% the 95% confidence intervals were 19% to 100%. This is a very wide range, within which the true benefit increase is estimated to lie. However, even the lowest estimate of 19% indicates clear benefit of the high-compression bandaging over the low-compression bandaging, and this is a statistically significant result.

In the text of their review, Cullum et al (2001) chose to express their results as relative risk, rather than odds ratios. However, as you will see from Table 7.4, what is demonstrated in the right-hand column is the odds ratio with 95% confidence interval. To obtain the odds ratio, the odds of complete healing in each group is first calculated. For the high-compression bandage group this is:

$$77/57 = 1.35$$

For the low-compression bandage group this is:

$$52/87 = 0.59$$

Therefore the odds ratio is:

$$1.35/0.60 = 2.26$$

Now look at the diagram in the fourth column. You will see a number of 'blobs' through which go horizontal lines. Reading the figures along the bottom axis, the point where the blob is represents the odds ratio for each individual trial. The horizontal line represents the 95% confidence interval of the individual trial. In this situation if both the odds ratio and the 95% confidence interval lie entirely to the right of the vertical line at 1 this means that there is a statistically significant benefit, in this case of elastic, high-compression stockings compared to inelastic, low-compression stockings, for the outcome being examined (complete healing of the ulcer in the trial period). If one looks at the three individual trials, it will be seen that this applies to only one trial (Cullum). In the other two trials (Gould and Northeast) the horizontal line crosses the vertical line of 1. This means that, although the odds ratio lies to the right of the line, the 95% confidence intervals include the line, so it is possible that the true result is 1 or even slightly less than 1 which means that there is no significant benefit. However, if the results from all three trials are combined the total result shown by the diamond at the bottom, where the 'blob' lies to the right of 1, indicates that the combined result is significant. The odds ratio of 2.26 suggests a large benefit of high-compression bandaging over low-compression bandaging. Cullum et al (2001) chose to express their results as relative risks rather than odds ratios, because their outcome of interest (complete ulcer healing) was not rare in either group. You will recall from the previous discussion that relative risks and odds ratios are only similar if the outcome is rare. They felt that to quote odds ratios would give an inflated impression of the magnitude of the effect.

How can systematic reviews inform practice?

Let us suppose that you are a practice nurse working in a busy inner city practice. There are high rates of unemployment and social deprivation within your practice population. You are concerned to find that three young men, all in their early 40s, have recently died from acute myocardial infarction. All three men were on your GP's list, but none had attended the surgery for the last 5 years. All were smokers.

These tragedies have prompted you to consider setting-up a 'well man clinic'. The aim of the clinic would be to identify men with risk factors for cardiovascular disease, and try to implement lifestyle changes which may reduce these risks. You plan to review all men on the practice list aged 40–60 in the first instance. Because of the large number of people that this will involve you will have a limited time for detailed discussions with each individual. You are in a dilemma about whether it would be appropriate to include specific counselling on smoking cessation for smokers who attend the clinic. You are not sure if they would take much notice of what you said anyway. You decide to look at the evidence for the effectiveness of advice from nurses on smoking cessation in this primary care setting.

You start by searching on the Cochrane Library. Using the advance search on NURS* AND (SMOKING AND CESSATION), restricted to the abstract, yields two systematic reviews in the Cochrane Database of Systematic Reviews. One of these, entitled 'Nursing interventions for smoking cessation' (Rice & Stead 2001) seems relevant to your question. A review of the 'criteria for considering studies' found that studies included were randomised trials in which adult smokers of either gender were recruited in any type of health care setting. The types of intervention included the provision of advice and/or other content and strategies to help patients quit smoking. The main outcome assessed was smoking cessation. The review group divided the interventions into low and high intensity for comparison. A low-intensity intervention was defined as trials where advice was provided (with or without a leaflet) during a single consultation lasting up to 10 minutes with up to one follow-up visit. High-intensity intervention was defined as trials where the initial contact lasted more than 10 minutes; there were additional materials (e.g. a manual) and/or strategies other than simple leaflets and the participants had more than one follow-up session. You were interested to look at the low-intensity comparison separately from the high-intensity comparison. This was because you knew your time would be limited and it would be feasible to spend up to 10 minutes with each man, provide a leaflet and see them for one follow-up visit, but you would not have the resources to do more than this.

The review included 22 trials. Five of these evaluated the 'low-intensity' intervention. These results are illustrated in Table 7.5. The pooled odds ratio for this group was, as you can see, 1.67 (95% CI 1.14–2.45). This was similar to the pooled odds ratio for

Table 7.5 **Nursing interventions for smoking cessation. The comparison shown is for low-intensity intervention versus control. The outcome is smoking cessation at longest follow-up**

Study	Expt n/N	Ctrl n/N	Peto OR (95%CI Fixed)	Weight %	Peto OR (95%CI Fixed)
Low-intensity intervention					
Davies 1992	2/153	4/154		0.8	0.51 [0.10,2.57]
Janz 1987	26/144	12/106		4.3	1.68 [0.84,3.38]
Nebot 1992	5/81	7/175		1.4	1.62 [0.47,5.63]
Tonnesen 1996	8/254	3/253		1.5	2.52 [0.76,8.31]
Vetter 1990	34/237	20/234		6.6	1.77 [1.00,3.12]
Subtotal (95% CI)	75/869	46/922		14.6	1.67 [1.14,2.45]
Chi-square 2.56 (df = 4) Z = 2.65					

.10 .20   1   5   10
Favours Control   Favours Treatment

Data from Cochrane Library (2001).

the 10 trials of high-intensity interventions, which was 1.47 (95% CI 1.26–1.72). You were concerned that a number of trials had evaluated nursing interventions for smoking cessation in hospitalised patients and you felt that the results might be better in that setting than in the clinic you were planning to set up. The analysis of all the studies, which looked at non-hospitalised patients, is shown in Table 7.6. This again showed an odds of success of well over 50% in the nursing intervention group compared with the control group (OR 1.81, 95% CI 1.39–2.36).

The quality of the review is appraised as described in Box 7.3. The objectives of the review clearly lay out the research question. A detailed search strategy has been prepared within the collaborative review group responsible for the review and this is comprehensive. Specific inclusion and exclusion criteria are reported and the quality of the included studies is clearly described. The meta-analysis addressed appropriate comparisons and was easy to understand. The conclusions of the review, which were that 'the results indicate potential benefits of smoking cessation advice counselling given by

Table 7.6 **Nursing interventions for smoking cessation. The comparison shown is for smoking intervention alone versus control in non-hospitalised patients. The outcome is smoking cessation at longest follow-up**

Study	Expt n/N	Ctrl n/N	Peto OR (95%CI Fixed)	Weight %	Peto OR (95%CI Fixed)
Smoking intervention alone in other non-hospitalized smokers					
Canga 2000	25/147	3/133	⟶	11.5	5.12 [2.35,11.17]
Davies 1992	2/153	4/154		2.7	0.51 [0.10,2.57]
Hollis 1993	79/1997	15/710		32.1	1.73 [1.09,2.77]
Janz 1987	26/144	12/106		14.4	1.68 [0.84,3.38]
Lancaster 1999	8/249	10/248		7.9	0.79 [0.31,2.03]
Nebot 1992	5/81	7/175		4.5	1.62 [0.47,5.63]
Tonnesen 1996	8/254	3/253		4.9	2.52 [0.76,8.31]
Vetter 1990	34/237	20/234		21.9	1.77 [1.00,3.12]
Subtotal (95%CI)	187/3262	74/2013		100.0	1.81 [1.39,2.36]
Chi-square 12.56					
(df = 7) Z = 4.40					

.10 .20   1   5   10

Favours Control   Favours Treatment

Data from Cochrane Library (2001).

nurses to their patients, with reasonable evidence that intervention can be effective', appear appropriate and supported by the evidence obtained in the review. You now feel very confident that introducing a smoking cessation strategy into your follow-up clinic for patients with risk factors for cardiovascular and respiratory disease will be effective and you are able to go ahead and plan the clinic.

It will be clear, by now, that systematic reviews are an important element of evidence-based practice. They are considered the 'gold standard' for assessing the effectiveness of a treatment or intervention. As a research activity they are important and need to be performed thoroughly. This chapter has described their basic methodology. All practitioners will need to use systematic reviews, so it is important to understand these methods and how the results are presented. They also need to be able to judge the quality of reviews to assess whether their results are valid.

References

Altman DG, Bland JM 1995 Absence of evidence is not evidence of absence. British Medical Journal 311: 485

Barnes D, Bero L 1998 Why review articles on the health effects of passive smoking reach different conclusions. Journal of the America Medical Association 279: 1566–1570

Bradley F, Field J 1995 Evidence-based medicine. Lancet 346: 838–839

Cochrane AL 1979 A critical review, with particular reference to the medical profession. In: Teeling-Smith G (ed) Medicines for the Year 2000. London: Office of Health Economics, pp 1931–1971

Cochrane Library 2001 The Cochrane Library, Disk Issue 3, 2001. Oxford: Update Software*

Crowley P 2001 Prophylactic corticosteroids for preterm birth (Cochrane Review). In: The Cochrane Library, Disk Issue 3, 2001. Oxford: Update Software

Cullum N, Nelson E, Fletcher A, Sheldon T 2001 Compression for venous leg ulcers (Cochrane Review). In: The Cochrane Library, Disk Issue 3, 2001. Oxford: Update Software*

Easterbrook PJ, Berlin JA, Gopalan R, Matthews DR 1991 Publication bias in clinical research. Lancet 337: 867–872

Jadad AR, Moher M, Browman G, Sigouin C, Fuentes M, Stevens R 2000 Systematic reviews and meta-analyses on treatment of asthma: critical evaluation. British Medical Journal 320: 537–540

Kalnins D, Durie P, Corey M, Ellis L, Pencharz P, Tullis E 1996 Are oral dietary supplements effective in the nutritional management of adolescents and adults with cystic fibrosis. Pediatric Pulmonology Suppl 13: 314–315*

Knipschild P 1995 Some examples of systematic reviews. In: Chalmers I, Altman DG (eds) Systematic Reviews. London: BMJ Publishing, 9–16

Linde K, Jobst K, Panton J 2001 Acupuncture for chronic asthma (Cochrane Review). In: The Cochrane Library, Disk Issue 3, 2001. Oxford: Update Software

Northeast A, Layer G, Wilson N, Browse N, Burnand K 1990 Increased compression expedites venous ulcer healing, Royal Society of Medicine Venous Forum

Oxman AD 1994 Checklists for review articles. British Medical Journal 309: 648–651

Pauling L 1986 How to live long and feel better. New York: Freeman

Poustie V, Watling R, Smyth RL 2001 Oral protein calorie supplementation for children with chronic disease (Cochrane Review). In: The Cochrane Library, Disk Issue 3, 2001. Oxford: Update Software*

Rice V, Stead L 2001 Nursing interventions for smoking cessation (Cochrane Review). In: The Cochrane Library, Disk Issue 3, 2001. Oxford: Update Software

---

*Cochrane Reviews are regularly updated as new information becomes available and in response to comments and criticisms. The reader should consult The Cochrane Library for the latest version of a Cochrane Review. Information on The Cochrane Library can be found at www.update-software.com.

Section 3

THE PROCESS OF CHANGING PRACTICE

8

Evidence-based guidelines

Lois Thomas and Rhona Hotchkiss

Key points

- The 1990s saw an unprecedented increase in guideline development activity in response to professional, public and political calls for evidence-based treatment delivered to comparable standards across the country.
- A potentially unlimited number of clinical topics may be amenable to guideline development. Criteria for topic selection have therefore had to be agreed.
- Rigorous methods are recommended for guideline development which is a time consuming, and often costly, process.
- Guidelines incorporate varying strengths of recommendation depending on the strength of the evidence they are based on.
- Instruments are available to appraise guidelines. These should be applied and the quality of the guideline judged before it is accepted for use.
- Strategies for the implementation of guidelines at local and individual clinician level must incorporate methods that have been demonstrated to be effective.

Introduction

Clinical guidelines are 'systematically developed statements to assist practitioner decisions about appropriate health care for specific clinical circumstances' (Field & Lohr 1990). The topic of a clinical guideline may be a condition (such as asthma or angina; North of England Evidence-Based Guideline Development Project 1999a, b), a symptom (such as pain; Royal College of Nursing 2000) or a clinical procedure (such as urinary catheter care; Seto et al 1991). Guidelines can be used to reduce inappropriate variations in practice and to promote the delivery of high-quality, evidence-based health care. They may also provide a mechanism by which health care professionals can be made accountable for clinical activities (Royal College of General Practitioners Clinical Guidelines Working Group 1995). While originally guidelines were based on consensus, individual opinion or both (and this remains the case in topics where there is little valid research evidence), it is now recognised that guidelines should be explicitly evidence-based. To date, most of the development and evaluation of clinical guidelines has been in medicine, but there is increasing interest in the use of guidelines in nursing (McClarey 1997, Royal College of Nursing 1995, Von Degenburg & Deighan 1995).

Guideline characteristics

If guidelines are to be effective, it is recommended that they have most, if not all, of the 11 characteristics listed in Box 8.1 (NHS Centre for Reviews and Dissemination (NHS CRD) 1994). Ensuring that guidelines meet these criteria is a resource-intensive task in terms of cost and the time and skills required both in developing evidence-based guidelines and in ensuring they remain up to date. The process from start of guideline development to publication has been estimated by the Scottish Intercollegiate Guidelines Network (SIGN 2001) to take up to 24 months, depending on the volume of relevant literature on the topic, the amount of feedback received during the consultation phase and the time constraints of the guideline development group. Guideline development may therefore be beyond the scope of practising health professionals, who may prefer to adopt or adapt guidelines developed nationally.

National or local guideline development

While locally developed ('internal') guidelines may need fewer resources and may be more likely to be adopted into clinical practice because of local ownership (Williamson 1978, Putnam & Curry 1985), local groups may not have the skills and resources required for guideline development (Grol 1990a, North of England Study of Standards and Performances in General Practice 1991). An alternative is the development of guidelines at regional/national level and subsequent modification to suit local circumstances (Grol 1990a, b, 1992).

Box 8.1 Characteristics of effective guidelines (NHS CRD 1994)

Attribute	Explanation
Validity	Evidence should be interpreted correctly so that if a guideline is followed, it leads to the predicted improvements in health
Cost-effectiveness	Improvements in health care should be at acceptable costs. If guidelines ignore issues of costs and concentrate only on benefits, there is the possibility that practices might be recommended with major implications for resource use which are not reflected in correspondingly large improvements in patient outcome
Reproducibility	Given the same evidence, another guideline development group would produce similar recommendations
Reliability	Given the same clinical circumstances another health professional would apply the recommendations in a similar fashion
Representative development	All key disciplines and interests contribute to guideline development
Clinical applicability	The target population is defined in accordance with the evidence
Clinical flexibility	Guidelines identify exceptions and indicate how patient preferences are to be incorporated into decision-making
Clarity	Guidelines use precise definitions, unambiguous language and user-friendly formats
Meticulous documentation	Guidelines record participants, assumptions and methods and link recommendations to the available evidence
Scheduled review	Guidelines state when and how they are to be reviewed
Utilisation review	Guidelines indicate ways in which adherence to recommendations can be sensibly monitored

Prioritising topic areas for guideline development

The NHS Executive in the UK suggested in 1996 that guideline development activity be targeted at clinical topics that include the following characteristics:

- Situations where there is evidence of excessive morbidity, disability or mortality.
- Conditions for which available treatment offers the potential for improvement in any of the above.
- Those where there is evidence of wide variation in practice.
- Conditions that are resource intensive either because they are high cost or high volume.
- Situations involving cross-boundary issues, for example interprofessional working or the need for joint working between primary and secondary care.

In this same document, the Executive makes the unequivocal statement that 'Clinical guidelines are produced for one reason, and one reason only: to improve the quality of care.' (page 7). However, in practice, other factors may dictate the guideline development agenda. Klein (1996) suggests that values, as opposed to research evidence, can determine the judgements made within 'guidelines', citing the example of the accessibility, or limits to the accessibility, of *in vitro* fertilisation treatment (IVF), where value-judgements are made about the ethics of individuals' situations.

Indeed the assertion that quality of care is the only factor to precipitate the development of a guideline is contradictory in the face of the criterion for development that concerns itself with resource-intensivity. Some of the earliest criticisms of or misgivings about guideline development arose because of cynicism around their purpose; that is, the suspicion that they could be an exercise in cost-containment.

The Scottish Intercollegiate Guidelines Network have a main criterion that there exists 'evidence of variation in practice which affects patient outcomes and a strong research base providing evidence of effective practice' (SIGN 2001). In addition, SIGN (2001) criteria for guideline development include:

- Conditions where effective treatment is proven and can reduce mortality or morbidity.

- Iatrogenic diseases/interventions where significant cost or risk is involved.
- Stated priority areas for the NHS in Scotland.

In a recent exercise designed to examine the priorities of nurses in Scotland for the development of 'Best Practice Statements' (www.nmpdu.org.uk), which will use scientific evidence, where it exists, combined with expert nursing opinion and consensus, topics that topped the poll were nutrition, continence, pressure ulcer prevention and others that many would consider 'basic' nursing care. Paradoxically, given the importance of these topics and the resources which their treatment costs the NHS, they have not been tackled by groups like SIGN. This may be because they lack sufficient evidence at the level of randomised controlled trial or well-conducted clinical trial prevalent in the topics that dominate the SIGN agenda. The prioritisation of topics for guideline development where recommendations are not open to wide dispute is understandable. However, the inevitable consequence of this is that matters that most concern nurses may fail to be prioritised.

How are guidelines developed?

Methods for developing evidence-based guidelines have been formalised both nationally (SIGN 2001) and locally (North of England Evidence Based Guideline Development Project 1999a, b). Recommended stages are similar and include:

- Selection of guideline topic
- Composition of the guideline development group
- Defining the scope of the guideline
- Systematic literature review
- Formation of recommendations
- Consultation and peer review
- Presentation and dissemination
- Local implementation
- Audit and review.

The guideline development group decides on the scope of the guideline, assesses available research evidence, and produces consensus recommendations which will aid practitioners in their health care decisions. According to SIGN (2001), four main skills are required in guideline development group members (but each member is not expected to have the full range):

1. Clinical expertise (e.g. nursing, physiotherapy, etc.)
2. Other specialist expertise (e.g. health economics, research methods)
3. Practical understanding of the problems faced in the delivery of care
4. Critical appraisal skills.

The group should ideally include representatives from all relevant disciplines and interested parties (Lomas 1993a), with representatives seeking the views of their colleagues to ensure that a balanced approach is taken. The optimum size for a group has been put at 8–10 (Scott 1990), but groups of between 10 and 20 members have been used successfully (SIGN 2001). A facilitator ensures that all members are free to contribute, that 'decibel level' does not determine priorities (Northern Regional Health Authority 1994), and that guideline recommendations accurately reflect the consensus of the whole group.

Patient involvement in guideline development

Patient involvement in their care is central to current government thinking (Department of Health 1997) and patient involvement in guideline development should be no exception. Patients' knowledge, understanding and experience of their illness makes them ideally placed to contribute, particularly in areas where guideline development is difficult because of lack of evidence. In the medical literature, however, patient involvement in guideline development groups is rare (van Wersch & Eccles 1999). Eccles et al (1996) invited a patient with asthma and a patient with stable angina to join the development group for the North of England Evidence Based Guidelines for asthma and angina respectively. However, the patients were described as 'non-participating observers' of technical discussions to which their contribution was minimal. Patients were not included in the guideline update team. The perceived difference in status between health professionals and patients may inhibit any constructive participation by patients, who may feel an uncomfortable minority (Bond & Grimshaw 1995).

Patients involved in guideline development groups have three potential roles (Box 8.2). Using a patient advocate may be one way

Box 8.2 Patient roles within guideline development groups

Title	Role
Patient	Presents their own views
Member of patient group	Presents the group's views
Patient advocate	Presents knowledge of patients' views

of increasing the likelihood of incorporating patients' views into guidelines and preventing the problems outlined above. It may be beneficial for the advocate (who is not a patient) to have:

- A broad knowledge of the subject of the guideline
- A knowledge of patients' experiences of coping with this symptom or condition
- An awareness of patients' feelings and problems
- An understanding of patients' needs
- Training in communication or counselling skills (Van Wersch & Eccles personal communication).

Soliciting patients' views outside the guideline development group and feeding these views back into group discussions may also be effective. This approach was used in the development of the guideline on the recognition and assessment of acute pain in children (Royal College of Nursing 2000): a qualitative study sought children's views and a children's conference was also held, where children described their experiences of pain through play, acting, drawing or interview (Doorbar & McClarey 1999). While anecdotal evidence suggests these approaches may be effective, there has been very little research into how best to use the patients' expertise in guideline development.

Once the group has been established, the scope of the guideline is defined. A number of key clinical questions are identified. A broad topic, for example the management of patients receiving chemotherapy, will take longer to develop and be more labour intensive than a topic that focuses on a single aspect of care such as mouthcare in children with cancer.

Next, a detailed literature search is conducted to look for evidence from research studies about the appropriateness and effectiveness of different clinical management strategies. Ideally, this will be a systematic review with defined inclusion and exclusion criteria, explicit criteria for assessing study quality, rigorous methods of data abstraction (for example data abstracted by two reviewers for each paper) and data synthesis. Although this approach demands a considerable amount of time and effort, applying scientific principles such as these to the review process reduces the risk of bias. Further information on systematic reviews is provided in Chapter 7.

Depending on the topic, the search strategy may include only certain study designs; for example, for the North of England Evidence Based Guidelines for the Management of Asthma (1996b) only randomised controlled trials, case control and cohort studies were searched for, while the guideline on the recognition and assessment of acute pain in children (Royal College of Nursing 2000), which was not concerned with the effectiveness of treatments, included a wider range of study designs.

A level of evidence is allocated to each paper, according to its methodological quality. Studies that have used an appropriate study design to address the research question, and are methodologically sound (for example, for a randomised controlled trial whether randomisation, allocation concealment, completeness of follow-up and intention to treat analysis have been adequately performed) are allocated a high level of evidence. The level is linked to the statement of evidence within the guideline: 'the administration of salbutamol using a large volume spacer with metered dose inhaler is as effective as nebulised salbutamol in patients with acute, but not life threatening, asthma. Level 1.'

The assigned level provides an indication of the potential for bias within the statement and is taken into consideration when recommendations are formulated. There are a number of interpretations of levels of evidence. Box 8.3 shows levels of evidence as defined by SIGN (SIGN 2001).

Next, the evidence is considered by the guideline development group and recommendations are formulated. This is a complex part of the process, especially where the evidence can be interpreted in a number of different ways. The guideline development group members are required to consider all of the evidence relating to each question, in the light of its methodological quality, and make recommendations that are explicitly based on the most robust evidence. Where recommendations vary, a process for reaching consensus is required. Recommendations are graded according to the level of evi-

---

Box 8.3 Statements of evidence (from SIGN 50, with kind permission of SIGN (Scottish Intercollegiate Guidelines Network)) © Scottish Intercollegiate Guidelines Network (SIGN), 2001.

1++ High-quality meta-analyses, systematic reviews of RCTs, or RCTs with a very low risk of bias

1+ Well-conducted meta-analyses, systematic reviews of RCTs, or RCTs with a low risk of bias

1 Meta-analyses, systematic reviews of RCTs, or RCTs with a high risk of bias

2++ High-quality systematic reviews of case control or cohort studies. High-quality case control or cohort studies with a very low risk of confounding, bias or chance and a high probability that the relationship is causal

2+ Well-conducted case control or cohort studies with a low risk of confounding, bias or chance and a moderate probability that the relationship is causal

2 Case control or cohort studies with a high risk of confounding, bias, or chance and a significant risk that the relationship is not causal

3 Non-analytic studies, e.g. case reports, case series

4 Expert opinion

---

dence, thus enabling readers to differentiate between those recommendations for which there is strong evidence and those based on weak evidence. Grading also enables guideline users to assess the predictive validity of each recommendation; recommendations based on strong evidence are more likely to achieve the predicted outcome (SIGN 2001). An example of grades of recommendation is shown in Box 8.4 (SIGN 2001).

Finally, the guideline is tested by asking professionals not involved in guideline development to review it for clarity, internal consistency and acceptability. The guideline can be piloted in selected health care settings to see whether its use is feasible in routine practice.

All guidelines should be reviewed after a specified time period to make sure they are updated to take into account new knowledge. Frequency of review will depend on the amount of new information in the particular topic area. If there have been significant

> **Box 8.4 Grades of recommendation from SIGN 50, with kind permission of SIGN (Scottish Intercollegiate Guidelines Network) © Scottish Intercollegiate Guidelines Network (SIGN) 2001.**
>
> A
> At least one meta analysis, systematic review, or RCT rated as I++, and directly applicable to the target population; or
> A systematic review of RCTs or a body of evidence consisting principally of studies rated as I+, directly applicable to the target population, and demonstrating overall consistency of results
>
> B
> A body of evidence including studies rated as 2++, directly applicable to the target population, and demonstrating overall consistency of results; or
> Extrapolated evidence from studies rated as I++ or I+
>
> C
> A body of evidence including studies rated as 2+, directly applicable to the target population and demonstrating overall consistency of results; or
> Extrapolated evidence from studies rated as 2++
>
> D
> Evidence level 3 or 4; or
> Extrapolated evidence from studies rated as 2+

developments in the evidence base, review may need to take place to incorporate these.

Consensus guidelines

If there is no high-quality research evidence to underpin all or some guideline recommendations, the views of a group of experts may be distilled through a consensus development process (Fink et al 1984). Achieving consensus is not easy and may be hampered by the most assertive or most authoritative group members having a greater say than others (Thomson et al 1995). There are, however, ways of getting the best out of a group, such as the Delphi technique or the nominal group technique (Jones & Hunter 1995). The

Delphi technique does not require group members to meet; instead group members generate topics of discussion. These are sent to all participants, who then comment in writing on their co-participants' views. Responses are analysed and collated and sent back to participants. The process continues until a consensus is reached.

The nominal group technique achieves consensus using highly structured meetings. It comprises two rounds in which participants rate, discuss and then re-rate a series of items or questions. The process is shown in Box 8.5.

The method can also be used within a single meeting and, in the context of guideline development, will include a detailed review of the literature as background material for the topic under discussion.

Example of an evidence-based guideline

The Royal College of Nursing is developing nurse-led guidelines in a number of areas. Examples include the management of venous leg ulcers and pressure ulcer risk assessment and prevention. The guideline for the recognition and assessment of acute pain in children was produced in 2000 and is described as 'evidence-linked', rather than evidence-based, as some recommendations are based on expert consensus opinion. The guideline includes a summary of graded recommendations for practice, as well as the rationale for each recommendation and a justification for each rating score. For this guideline, a simple grading system (Box 8.6) was used.

Box 8.5 Stages in the nominal group technique (Jones & Hunter 1995)

- Participants write down their views on topic in question
- Each participant, in turn, contributes one idea to the facilitator, who records it on a flip chart
- Similar suggestions are grouped together where appropriate. There is group discussion to clarify and evaluate each idea
- Each participant privately ranks each idea
- The ranking is tabulated and presented
- The overall ranking is discussed and re-ranked
- Final rankings are tabulated and results fed back to participants

Box 8.6 Grades of recommendation used in the guideline The recognition and assessment of acute pain in children (Royal College of Nursing 2000, with permission)

Grade I

Generally consistent finding in a majority of multiple acceptable studies

Grade II

Either based on a single acceptable study, or a weak or inconsistent finding in multiple acceptable studies

Grade III

Limited scientific evidence which does not meet all the criteria of acceptable studies or absence of directly applicable studies of good quality. This includes published and unpublished expert opinion.

An example showing a range of recommendations is given in Box 8.7.

Appraising published guidelines

Developing new evidence-based guidelines is expensive and time-consuming and it is therefore preferable, in the majority of cases, to use previously published guidelines if these are applicable and of good quality. Some useful websites for finding guidelines are given at the end of this chapter. A validated UK instrument is available for appraising the quality of published guidelines (Cluzeau et al 1997). Areas covered are shown in Box 8.8.

While using this tool will give a good indication of guideline quality, it is likely that many will not score highly on all sections of the instrument because of lack of documentation on the process of guideline development (Thomson et al 1995).

Adapting nationally developed guidelines for local use

The translation of nationally developed or other guidelines developed 'externally' into protocols for local use is both per-

> **Box 8.7 Example of recommendations for the recognition and assessment of acute pain in children (Royal College of Nursing 2000, with permission)**
>
> **2 Indicators of children's pain**
>
> 2.1 Note changes in children's behaviour, appearance, activity level and vital signs as these may indicate a change in the pain intensity — Grade I
>
> 2.2 Use physiological measures (e.g. heart and respiratory rates) but only in addition to self-report and behavioural measures to determine whether children are in pain — Grade II
>
> **3 Individual differences**
>
> 3.1 Obtain a patient history from each child and his/her parents at the time of admission and learn what word the child uses for pain (e.g. hurt, baddie, etc.) — Grade II
>
> 3.2 Recognise the importance of and seek to identify cultural factors which may affect the assessment of pain — Grade III

missible and, in the opinion of many commentators, desirable. Feder et al (1999) suggest that, just as topics for guideline development require to be prioritised against a set of accepted criteria, so local organisations must develop a system for prioritising the implementation of guidelines locally. The sheer volume of recommendations contained within all of the clinical guidelines that might be applicable to the work of a general practitioner in the NHS, for example, make prioritising according to local need a necessity. The SIGN organisation has now produced in excess of 20 guidelines whose recommendations have implications for general practice; SIGN is only one such organisation among many.

Local adaptation of guidelines also has the potential for mitigating some of the objections to their use detailed below; for example, that they may lack local relevance. Asking local clinical teams to appraise 'external' guidelines and prioritise their implementation may also bring a sense of ownership that can be difficult to achieve otherwise.

Box 8.8 Areas covered by Appraisal Instrument for Clinical Guidelines (Cluzeau et al 1997, with permission from St George's Hospital Medical School, London)

Topic	Example
Dimension 1: Rigour of development	
Responsibility for guideline development	Is the agency responsible for guideline development clearly identified?
Guideline development group	Is there a description of individuals who were involved in the guidelines development group?
Identification and interpretation of evidence	Is there a description of the method(s) used to interpret and assess the strength of evidence?
Formulation of recommendations	Is there a description of methods used to formulate the recommendations?
Peer review	Were the guidelines independently reviewed prior to their publication/release?
Updating	Is there mention of a date for reviewing or updating the guidelines?
Overall assessment of the development process	Overall, have the potential biases of guideline development been dealt with?
Dimension 2: Context and content	
Objectives	Are the reasons for developing the guidelines clearly stated?
Context	Is there a satisfactory description of the patients to which the guidelines are meant to apply?
Clarity	Do the guidelines describe the condition to be detected, treated, or prevented in unambiguous terms?

Likely costs and benefits	Is there an adequate description of the health benefits that are likely to be gained from the recommended management?
Dimension 3: Application	
Guideline dissemination and implementation	Does the guideline document suggest possible methods for dissemination and implementation?
Monitoring of guidelines/ clinical audit	Does the guideline document specify criteria for monitoring compliance?
National guidelines only	Does the guideline document identify key elements which need to be considered by local guideline groups?

Issues of resource availability and potential returns in terms of health gain also need to be considered. This, though, raises the issue of when local adaptation becomes unacceptable, potentially recreating the situation guidelines are designed to address. The National Institute of Clinical Excellence (NICE) in England has recently issued guidance on the use of beta-interferon for people with multiple sclerosis and has made a judgement against its use. Had they decided for its use, it may have had little effect on the budgets of some Health Authorities/Boards in areas of low incidence, whilst in other areas such as the South West of Scotland where there is a higher than average incidence of multiple sclerosis, the costs would have been high and would arguably have meant that other services could have suffered as a result. Interestingly, Hurwitz (1999) suggests that 'users of guidelines are expected to behave as learned intermediaries, exercising customary clinical discretion and consulting other sources of relevant information.'

Patient versions of guidelines

Versions of guidelines which patients can understand and which are written in their own language are considered essential by NICE.

While there are patient versions available, for example of the Inter-collegiate National Clinical Guidelines on Stroke (Intercollegiate Working Party for Stroke 2000) and the Recognition and Assessment of Acute Pain in Children (Royal College of Nursing 2000) there has been little research into the effectiveness of these and what their role is in providing information or helping patients manage their condition.

Introducing the guideline into practice

Once a clinical guideline is ready for use, there are two stages which facilitate its introduction into practice: dissemination and implementation. Dissemination is generally taken to refer to the method by which the guidelines are made available to potential users. Strategies include publication in professional journals and sending the guideline to targeted individuals, as well as strategies involving an educational intervention. Several studies have assessed the effectiveness of different strategies: dissemination by publication or direct mailing have been found to be the least successful (Freemantle et al 2001, Grol 1992, Lomas et al 1989), but have the advantage of being cheap and reproducible. Strategies involving an educational component, especially where this is specifically targeted rather than in the form of continuing education, are more likely to result in behaviour change (Lomas et al 1991). However, dissemination alone without an appropriate implementation strategy is unlikely to influence behaviour significantly (Grimshaw et al 1995).

Implementation is a means of ensuring that users subsequently act upon the recommendations. 'Implementation is a more active process, involving tailoring the message to the needs of the target audience, and actively working to overcome barriers to behaviour change' (Lomas 1993b). Implementation strategies try to ensure that users adopt and apply guidelines to which they have access. Grol (1992) suggests that in designing an implementation strategy it is necessary to be aware of barriers to behaviour change; these may include both structural and attitudinal factors and appropriate interventions might be targeted at both the structure and the process of care. Some implementation strategies supply accessible reminders of the guideline. For example, patient-specific prompts at the time of consultation are thought to be a powerful strategy (Emslie et al 1993, Grimshaw & Russell 1993, Lilford et al 1992).

Audit and feedback has also been shown to be capable of affecting doctors' behaviour: a systematic review of randomised controlled trials found effects to be small, but potentially worthwhile (Thomson-O'Brien et al 2001).

Evaluating the effectiveness of clinical guidelines in nursing and professions allied to medicine

Most of the literature on clinical guidelines comes from medicine. However, a recent systematic review for the Cochrane Collaboration examined whether clinical guidelines are effective in changing the behaviour of nurses, midwives and health visitors and other professions allied to medicine (Thomas et al 1998, 2001). Key points are summarised in Box 8.9. Eighteen evaluations of guidelines were found; all but one of these studies evaluated the introduction of guidelines targeting nurses. Guidelines evaluated included the management of urinary catheter care (Seto et al 1991), hypertension (Jewell & Hope 1988), and postoperative bleeding after cardiac surgery (Zeler et al 1992).

Box 8.9 Key points from systematic review of the effectiveness of clinical guidelines in nursing, midwifery and professions allied to medicine (Thomas et al 1998, 2001)

- Significant changes in some processes of care were found in four out of five studies measuring process

- Six out of eight studies measuring outcomes found significant differences favouring the group who received guidelines

- Three studies evaluated dissemination and implementation strategies: findings appear to suggest that educational interventions (e.g. lectures, teaching sessions) are of more value than passive approaches (e.g. postal distribution) in the dissemination of guidelines, however methodological flaws limit the credibility of findings

- Studies examining the ability of guidelines to enable skill substitution generally support the hypothesis of no difference between nurse-protocol driven and physician care

While this review has provided some evidence that guideline-driven care can be effective in changing the practice of nurses and patient outcomes, there is a long way to go before guidelines meeting the 11 criteria (Box 8.1, page 189) are routinely used by nurses to improve patient care. While all guidelines should be underpinned by evidence of effectiveness, reports of the guideline development process in studies included in the review typically contained scant details of the methods used for identifying and assessing relevant evidence. Although many of the guidelines identified were based on a literature review, the extent to which these reviews were systematic was not described, nor were the quality criteria by which any evidence was assessed. This calls into question the validity of the guidelines and their consequent potential for patient benefit. Guidelines produced by the Royal College of Nursing (1998, 2000) have been rigorously developed but need to be evaluated to see if they are effective in changing professional behaviour and patient outcomes.

Benefits and disbenefits of clinical guidelines

Clinical guidelines, integrated care pathways, protocols of care and any other externally imposed directive pertaining to treatment and intervention with patients will arguably all face the same set of objections, misconceptions and concerns about their use and, importantly, their legal standing as discussed below. 'Externally imposed' in relation to clinical care might be understood to be any directive about a clinician's action, the devising of which any individual clinician may not have been involved in.

Objections to, and support for, the use of guidelines are based on differing perceptions of the problems they are designed to address and of the related benefits or disbenefits they bring.

The use of guidelines has been criticised on the grounds that they can:

- Stifle individual clinical judgement
- De-skill professionals by reducing their capacity to think for themselves
- Limit quality of care by restricting care/treatment options
- Introduce practice which could be ineffective or dangerous
- Encourage the illusion that there is clear-cut direction to be taken in every clinical situation

- Be very resource-intensive in relation to their development and implementation
- Lack local relevance
- Concentrate on 'easy' areas, that is where there is already a body of evidence about appropriate treatment
- Allow powerful and vocal individuals to impose their priorities on particular services
- Require clinicians to follow courses of action for which they do not have the requisite skills or knowledge
- Raise patient expectations about types and standards of care they might expect to receive.

For each of these criticisms or objections there is an opposing assertion or opinion. It has been suggested that guidelines:

- Ensure safe practice
- Improve consistency of care in different parts of the country/settings of care
- Make it more likely that patients receive correct treatment
- Build parity of knowledge amongst staff
- Bring the expert opinion to everyday clinical care
- Allow for individual patient variation – non-application is not disallowed, it simply has to be justified
- Provide more information for patients about what they should expect from the health care system
- Distill the vast array of knowledge relating to individual clinical conditions into a manageable guide for busy clinicians
- Allow room for the development of local protocols.

The restriction of individual clinical judgement and the apparent requirement to treat all patients the same, regardless of individual idiosyncrasies or characteristics, seems to be at the heart of most objections to or difficulties with the use of guidelines. Likewise the heart of the defence case for the use of guidelines seems to be the argument that patients deserve the best possible treatment all of the time in definable situations regardless of the individual expertise of the person dealing with them at the time; if guidelines can expedite that best treatment, the argument goes, then they have a legitimate place in the system.

The acid test for clinical guidelines and the answer to any criticisms would surely proceed from proof of their benefit to patient care. As outlined above, more studies are needed to assess the impact of guideline development.

Conclusion

If guidelines are to be underpinned by evidence of effective practice, a prerequisite is high-quality evidence of the benefits and costs of the procedures and practices targeted. Further research into the effectiveness of nursing practice and interventions is required in order to provide this evidence base. Particular attention should be given to the provision of high-grade evidence from randomised controlled trials, rather than from weaker quasi-experimental designs, where the research question allows this approach.

Nurses whose behaviour is targeted by guidelines need to have an active role in their development or adaptation to local circumstances: this approach will encourage 'ownership' of the guideline and is more likely to lead to more positive attitudes towards it. It will also ensure that profession-specific practices and barriers and facilitating factors in bringing about behaviour change are taken into account.

Where possible, the introduction of clinical guidelines should be within an evaluative framework: nursing requires more evidence that those dissemination and implementation strategies which have proved to be most effective in changing doctors' behaviour are effective in changing the behaviour of nurses.

Clinical guidelines are a potential means by which evidence can be incorporated into nursing practice. However, more research is clearly required into the most effective ways of developing, disseminating and implementing clinical guidelines in nursing. Only then will a decision be possible about their potential for improving nursing practice and patient outcomes.

References

Bond CM, Grimshaw JM 1995 Multi-disciplinary guideline development: a case study from community pharmacy. Health Bulletin 53: 26–33

Cluzeau F, Littlejohns P, Grimshaw J, Feder G 1997 Appraisal instrument for clinical guidelines. London: St George's Hospital Medical School

Department of Health 1997 The new NHS: modern, dependable. London: Department of Health

Doorbar P, McClarey M 1999 Ouch! sort it out: children's experiences of pain. London: RCN Publishing

Eccles MP, Clapp Z, Grimshaw J et al 1996 Developing valid guidelines: methodological and procedural issues from the North of England evidence based guideline development project. Quality in Health Care 5: 44–50

Emslie CJ, Grimshaw J, Templeton A 1993 Do clinical guidelines improve general practice management and referral of infertile couples? British Medical Journal 306: 1728–1731

Feder G, Eccles M, Grol R, Griffiths C, Grimshaw J 1999 Using clinical guidelines. British Medical Journal 318(7185): 728–730

Field MJ, Lohr KN 1990 Clinical practice guidelines: directions for a new program. Washington DC: National Academy Press

Fink A, Kosecoff J, Chassin M, Brook RH 1984 Consensus methods: characteristics and guidelines for use. American Journal of Public Health 74(9): 979–983

Freemantle N, Harvey EL, Wolf F, Grimshaw JM, Grilli R, Bero LA 2001 Printed educational materials to improve the behaviour of health care professionals and patient outcomes (Cochrane Review). In: The Cochrane Library, Issue 3, 2001. Oxford: Update Software

Grimshaw J, Russell IT 1993 Effect of clinical guidelines on medical practice: a systematic review of rigorous evaluations. Lancet 342: 1317–1322

Grimshaw J, Freemantle N, Wallace S et al 1995 Developing and implementing clinical practice guidelines. Quality in Health Care 4: 55–64

Grol R 1990a National standard setting for quality of care in general practice: attitudes of general practitioners and response to a set of standards. British Journal of General Practice 40: 361–364

Grol, R 1990b Quality assurance: approaches to standard setting, assessment and change. Atencion Primaria (Barcelona) 7: 737–741

Grol R 1992 Implementing guidelines in general practice care. Quality in Health Care 184–191

Hurwitz B 1999 Legal and political considerations of clinical practice guidelines. British Medical Journal 318(7184): 661–664

Intercollegiate Working Party for Stroke 2000 Care after stroke: information for patients and their carers. London: Royal College of Physicians

Jewell D, Hope J 1988 Evaluation of a nurse-run hypertension clinic in general practice. Practitioner 232: 484–487

Jones J, Hunter D 1995 Consensus methods for medical and health services research. British Medical Journal 311: 376–380

Klein R 1996 The NHS and the new scientism: solution or delusion? Quarterly Journal of Medicine 89:85–87

Lilford RJ, Kelly M, Baines A et al 1992 Effect of using protocols on medical care: randomised trial of three methods of taking an antenatal history. British Medical Journal 305: 1181–1184

Lomas J 1993a Making clinical policy explicit. Legislative policy making and lessons for developing practice guidelines. International Journal of Technology Assessment in Health Care 9: 11–25

Lomas J 1993b Teaching old (and not so old) docs new tricks: effective ways to implement research findings, Working paper 93–4. Toronto: McMaster University Centre for Health Economics and Policy Analysis

Lomas J, Anderson G, Pierre K, Vayda E, Enkin M, Hannah W 1989 Do practice guidelines guide practice? The effect of a consensus statement on the practice of physicians. New England Journal of Medicine 321: 1306–1311

Lomas J, Enkin M, Anderson GM, Hannah WJ, Vayda E, Singer J 1991 Opinion leaders vs audit and feedback to implement practice guidelines. Delivery after previous cesarean section. Journal of the American Medical Association 265(17): 2202–2207

McClarey M 1997 Identifying priorities for guideline development as a result of nursing needs. DQI Network News 6: 4–5

NHS Centre for Reviews and Dissemination 1994 Implementing clinical practice guidelines. Leeds: University of Leeds

NHS Executive 1996 Clinical guidelines. Using clinical guidelines to improve patient care within the NHS. National Health Service Management Executive, Leeds

North of England Evidence Based Guideline Development Project 1999a The primary care management of stable angina. Newcastle upon Tyne: Centre for Health Services Research

North of England Evidence Based Guideline Development Project 1999b The primary care management of asthma in adults. Newcastle upon Tyne: Centre for Health Services Research

North of England Study of Standards and Performances in General Practice 1991 Overview of the study. Newcastle upon Tyne: Centre for Health Services Research

Northern Regional Health Authority 1994 Guidelines – a resource pack. Newcastle upon Tyne, pp 1–40

Putnam RW, Curry L 1985 Impact of patient care appraisal on physician behaviour in the office setting. Canadian Medical Association Journal 132: 1025–1029

Royal College of General Practitioners Clinical Guidelines Working Group 1995 The development and implementation of clinical guidelines. London: Royal College of General Practitioners

Royal College of Nursing 1995 Clinical guidelines: what you need to know. London: Royal College of Nursing

Royal College of Nursing 1998 The management of patients with venous leg ulcers. London: RCN Publishing

Royal College of Nursing 2000 The recognition and assessment of acute pain in children. London: Royal College of Nursing

Scott M, Marinker ML 1990 Medical audit and general practice. London: British Medical Journal

Seto WH, Ching TY, Yuen KY, Chu YB, Seto WL 1991 The enhancement of infection control in-service education by ward opinion leaders. American Journal of Infection Control 19: 86–91

SIGN (Scottish Intercollegiate Guidelines Network) 2001 A guideline developers' handbook. SIGN publication no. 50 (http://www.sign.ac.uk/guidelines/fulltext/50/)

Thomas LH, McColl E, Cullum N, Rousseau N, Soutter J, Steen N 1998 Effect of clinical guidelines in nursing, midwifery and the therapies: a systematic review of evaluations. Quality in Health Care 7: 183–191

Thomas LH, McColl E, Cullum N, Rousseau N, Soutter J, Steen N 2001 Systematic review of the effectiveness of clinical guidelines in nursing, midwifery and professions allied to medicine (Cochrane Review). In: The Cochrane Library, Issue 4. Oxford: Update Software

Thomson R, Lavender M, Madhok R 1995 How to ensure that guidelines are effective. British Medical Journal 311: 237–242

Thomson-O'Brien MA, Oxman AD, Davis DA, Haynes RB, Freemantle N, Harvey EL 2001 Audit and feedback to improve health professional practice and health care outcomes (Cochrane Review). In: The Cochrane Library, Issue 1. Oxford: Update Software

Van Wersch A, Eccles M 1999 Patient involvement in evidence-based health in relation to clinical guidelines. In: Gabbay M (ed) The evidence-based primary care handbook. London: Royal Society of Medicine Press, pp 91–103

Von Degenberg K, Deighan M 1995 Guideline development: A model of multi-professional collaboration. In: Deighan M, Hitch S (eds) Clinical effectiveness from guidelines to cost-effective practice. London: Department of Health, pp 93–97

Williamson JW 1978 Formulating priorities for quality assurance activity. Description of a method and its application. Journal of the American Medical Association 239: 631–637

Zeler KM, McPharlane TJ, Salamonsen RF 1992 Effectiveness of nursing involvement in bedside monitoring and control of coagulation status after cardiac surgery. American Journal of Critical Care 1: 70–75

Further reading

Thomas LH, McColl E, Cullum N, Rousseau N, Soutter J, Steen N 2001 Systematic review of the effectiveness of clinical guidelines in nursing, midwifery and professions allied to medicine (Cochrane Review). In: The Cochrane Library, Issue 4. Oxford: Update Software
This Cochrane Review examines the effectiveness of clinical guidelines in changing professional behaviour and patient outcomes in nursing, midwifery and professions allied to medicine.

Thomas LH, McColl E, Cullum N, Rousseau N, Soutter J 1999 Clinical guidelines in nursing, midwifery and the therapies: a systematic review. Journal of Advanced Nursing 30(1): 40–50
This paper describes the characteristics of guidelines evaluated and the effectiveness of different dissemination and implementation strategies used.

Appendix 8.1
Useful websites

The National Institute for Clinical Effectiveness
http://www.nice.org.uk/nice-web/

The Royal College of Nursing (RCN clinical guidelines can be accessed from this site)
http://www.rcn.org.uk/services/promote/clinical/clinical_guidelines.htm/

Scottish Intercollegiate Guidelines Network
http://www.show.scot.nhs.uk/sign/guidelines/

National Electronic Library for Health guidelines database
http://www.nelh.nhs.uk/guidelines_database.asp

Agency for Healthcare Research and Quality
http://www.ahcpr.gov/

9

How can we develop an evidence-based culture?

Carl Thompson and Mark Learmonth

Key points

- The national policy imperative
- The shape of culture generally and evidence-based culture specifically
- Potential barriers to cultural change
- The need for diagnosis, planning and marketing
- What works and what does not work in changing behaviours
- Real life examples.

Introduction

Culture shapes the beliefs and behaviours of people in the workplace. Without an awareness of the impact of culture on the implementation and utilisation of research evidence then strategies for change will almost certainly fail. Changing culture, however, is like juggling jelly: more than a little problematic (Davies et al 2000, Parker 2000), and a degree of realism needs to be fostered and maintained. Our aim in writing this chapter is to provide raw materials that organisational managers (and clinicians) might like to consider using when developing successful real world, realistic strategies for evidence-based change in their organisations.

The national picture

In the late 1990s, the UK government pursued a systematic approach to quality improvement in the National Health Service (NHS). Clinical governance (Secretary of State for Health 1998) is the term intended to encapsulate this approach – officially defined as:

a framework through which NHS organisations are accountable for continuously improving the quality of their services and safeguarding high standards of care by creating an environment in which excellence in clinical care will flourish. (Secretary of State for Health 1998, page 33)

The Boards of NHS organisations now have a formal duty to ensure that quality is improved and new bodies, such as the National Institute for Clinical Excellence (NICE), National Service Frameworks (NSF), and the Commission for Health Improvement (CHI), have been established in order to assist this process (Figure 9.1). The functions of these and other national bodies are discussed in detail in Chapter 11. Poor practice will be ever less acceptable. Chief executives will be subject to audit of the overall performance of their organisation (Secretary of State for Health 2000) and they are likely, therefore, increasingly to scrutinise the quality of health care provision in individual clinical areas. The question 'How can we develop an evidence-based practice culture?' is set to become increasingly pertinent.

What does an evidence-based culture look like?

Organisational culture generally

Organisational culture can be seen as the totality of social interactions that take place in work settings (Calas and Smircich 1987).

Figure 9.1 **The NHS quality structure (from Department of Health 1998 with permission)**

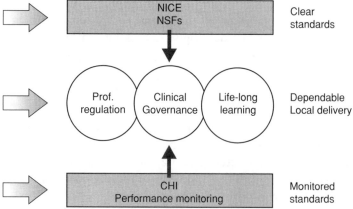

Because culture is all encompassing, leaders or managers are as much part of the culture as everyone else, rather than being able to 'stand outside' and manipulate it. Culture is a complex entity and given this truism the reader should recognise that easy 'fixes' are not a realistic option. For a discussion of the complexities of culture, readers are directed to the texts offered by Parker (2000) and Gabriel (1999). If culture then is an umbrella term for all social interactions in a hospital, clinic or service, where should the clinician look to focus their efforts at change? Indeed, is there such an entity as an evidence-based practice culture at all?

An evidence-based practice culture

Muir Gray (1997) suggests that the basis for health care provision rests on the decisions made within its structures and organisations. An evidence-based practice culture is one in which more good decisions are made than bad, and where research evidence, patient preferences, the available resources and clinical expertise, play an active part in decision-making processes (DiCenso et al 1998, Sackett et al 2000) (Figure 9.2).

The key components of an evidence-based organisation then are 'a built in...capability to generate, and the flexibility to incor-

Figure 9.2 An evidence-based health care decision

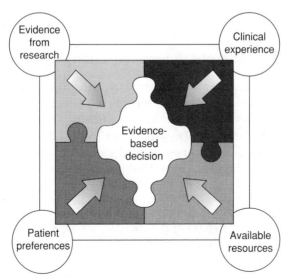

porate, evidence and individuals and teams who can find, appraise and use research evidence' (Muir Gray 1997, page 155). In order to achieve these characteristics the organisation is dependent on the cultures, systems and structures contained within it. Moreover, each of these elements shares a degree of interdependence: systems that promote evidence-based decisions are no use unless accompanied by supportive structures and a facilitative cultural environment.

The process of evidence-based health care is based around five key stages:

1. converting health care problems into focused health care questions
2. searching for the best available research evidence
3. critically appraising the evidence retrieved
4. implementing the evidence
5. auditing the implementation.

Evidence-based organisational culture is one in which individuals and groups (and the systems and structures they develop) are totally committed to each of these stages and at all organisational levels. As Brown (1999) notes, an organisational culture for evidence-based health care requires obsessional commitment at the level of the individual, clinical teams or practice groups, and health care systems and organisations.

Diagnosing the challenges to changing practice

Because of the complexities involved in changing cultures, it is generally accepted that in order to introduce evidence into practice, a diagnosis needs to be made of the challenges faced. The NHS Centre for Reviews and Dissemination (NHS CRD) in their systematic overview of interventions designed to influence professional behaviour (NHS CRD 1999) suggest that such diagnosis should include:

- identifying all the groups involved in, affected by, or influencing the proposed change(s) in practice
- assessing the characteristics of the proposed change that might influence its adoption
- assessing the preparedness of the health professionals to change

and other potentially relevant internal factors within the target group

- identifying the potential external barriers to change
- identifying the likely enabling factors, including resources and skills.

A variety of methods exist for gaining a purchase on these categories, but possible options include:

- Surveying key groups of stakeholders (such as senior staff, managers, and patient representatives): this could include auditing existing resources to identify staff with significant research appraisal and change management skills.

- Adapting ward meetings or clinical supervision sessions so that potential problems can be identified, recorded and fed into the strategic planning process.

- Establishing a focus group of professionals, managers and, where appropriate, patient representatives, to identify pertinent barriers and drivers. Cameron and Wren (1999) used this approach by forming 'buzz' groups of six to eight people who used 'reflection-on-action' (Schon 1983) to identify their values. These were typed and distributed to the group under the heading 'organizational values'. Efforts were made within the group to ensure that a collective understanding of the values identified was achieved.

- Isolating some of the barriers to research uptake in clinical practice. The 'Barriers Scale' (Funk et al 1991) builds on the recognition that barriers to research utilisation occur at various levels. These include: the values, skills and awareness of the practitioner wishing to use research, the barriers and limitations associated with the organisation, the qualities or characteristics of the research itself, and the ways in which research is presented and made accessible (or not). This scale has been used in a number of studies and could provide a useful tool for those wishing to identify some of the likely blocks in their environment (Dunn et al 1998, Nilson Kajermo et al 1998, Parahoo 2000, Retsas 2000) but its standing as a diagnostic tool has not been established. It is probably best considered as part of a multifaceted approach to planning for evidence-based intervention.

Common complexities associated with nursing and research use

Whilst individual practice environments will always be different there are four main groups of variables (or management challenges) which anyone considering changes in a health service environment may wish to consider: professional cultural, information related, environmental and individual.

Professional cultural

Evidence-based health care is about matching the most appropriate evidence to the clinical question being asked. Sometimes this will merit qualitative research and sometimes quantitative. Nurse leaders, educators and opinion formers need to recognise that some forms of research evidence are better at answering some forms of clinical questions than others (even those that nursing has traditionally not been involved in, such as the randomised controlled trial) and that practitioners should be encouraged to remain open-minded. A fear of quantitative approaches can mean that practitioners shy away from studies with 'lots of statistics' and construct or frame problems in ways which lead to more qualitative solutions. Our own studies at York reveal that the sorts of questions nurses raise in practice do, indeed, merit quantitative research evidence. For example, 'Which dressing best promotes healing?' or 'What is the increase in risk of another heart attack in my patient with diabetes?' But this in no way undermines the importance of qualitative research evidence where relevant. Nurses have unique insights into patients' beliefs and behaviours and such information is invaluable in informing much of nursing practice.

Nurses should be encouraged to match the information they look for to the kinds of questions they need answers to, rather than constructing questions around sources of information with which they feel comfortable. Opinion and clinical leaders, educators, Research and Development support, and practice development staff should lead by example and take responsibility for developing the necessary skills and knowledge in practitioners. Indeed, one of the common views of nurses we interviewed was that their experience of being introduced to statistics as a student nurse deterred them from engaging with quantitative research for the rest of their career. The current fashion of problem-based approaches to educating nurses (coupled with an awareness on the part of educators of the potential of quantitative research evidence) should encourage greater contact with these approaches. Indeed, it is difficult to know how a nurse faced with a mother who wants to know what the risks of immunisation are, or a middle-aged man who wants to know the implications of a positive test result when screened for prostate cancer, would react if they only accessed qualitative research in response to their clinical uncertainty.

Information related

The structure, volume and nature of clinical information available to nurses, and the provision of relevant training, are key indicators of a serious organisational commitment to evidence-based health care. Many of the resources available to nurses are not particularly suited to evidence-based practice. Some recent research at the University of York (Thompson et al 2000) revealed that in three large acute hospital trusts (which previous research had shown were more likely to have access to up-to-date materials and resources) the written materials that nurses had access to were:

- out of date (average age of more than 5 years)
- not evidence-based: only around a quarter of journal articles were reports of studies or literature reviews with explicit references to research. Only 13% of the guidelines or protocols had any explicit research base
- variable across clinical domains (coronary care had more evidence-based resources than general medical or surgical units)
- poorly organised, with no central means of establishing what resources actually exist
- concerned with 'background knowledge' in the form of anatomy or physiology rather than giving clues as to the management (foreground knowledge) of patient problems.

Good-quality information has to be fit for the purposes of reducing the uncertainty associated with clinical decision-making, and organisations/individual units need to consider the fitness for purpose of their literature and information resources. In the case of health care information, less is often more; i.e. less volume but higher quality information matched to the specific needs of the clinical area may prove more useful than a shelf of ageing textbooks. High-quality text-based resources which synthesize the results of primary or secondary research (such as the journals *Evidence Based Nursing* or *Evidence Based Mental Health*), together with library access and on-line searching and storage facilities should be the goal of every ward or unit.

The shape and format of the formal and informal continuing professional development should also be considered. Teaching sessions and initiatives such as journal clubs and study days could be adapted so that information retrieval is linked to the development and posing of clinical questions (based on real life clinical problems). This will help to highlight the resource requirements for reducing uncertainty. Moreover the training of staff in the use of resources such as the Cochrane Library, Best Evidence, CINAHL or MEDLINE will be that much more meaningful if it uses ward- or clinic-based technology and real life problems and decisions.

Environmental

Nurses working in different specialties, for example coronary care units (CCUs) compared with the community, or nurses with different levels of expertise (Crow et al 1995, Jacavone & Dostal 1992, White et al 1992) may handle similar decisions very differently. Clinical domains limit or shape the choices and hypotheses associated with clinical decisions. The point here is that solutions developed in one setting or with one organisational group may not be directly transferable to another health care environment (for example, acute secondary care to primary care) or group. Of course, diagnosing the challenges that are specific to each subgroup will highlight essential areas of focus and so is a key stage of any planned change intervention.

Different clinical domains also have varying amounts of good-quality research evidence. For example, nurses responsible for wound care have a large selection of randomised controlled trials and published systematic reviews of these trials to act as data for informing their decisions, while those in urology are not so well served. In these areas it is clear that organisations have to rely on the best available evidence. Where this evidence cannot come from research, then alternatives might include the development of local consensus technologies such as clinical guidelines coupled with the auditing of outcomes which are clinically significant.

A supportive professional and administrative environment significantly influences the use of research-based evidence (Funk et al

1995). Nilson Kajermo and colleagues (1998, 2000) found that characteristics of support included: interest, devotion, professional pride, a sympathetic attitude to research, courage and willingness to carry out changes. Moreover, a supportive administrative environment is associated with satisfaction among the workforce, which itself has been shown to be a positive correlate for adoption of research-based practice (Coyle & Sokow 1990).

Individual decision-maker

The environmental factors outlined above are complemented by a number of variables located at the level of the individual. Interestingly, there is little reliable evidence to suggest that the age and experience of a workforce are associated with increased research utilisation. There are, however, some variables which the organisation can influence.

Knowledge and educational attainment

Studies using proxy indicators for knowledge (such as educational attainment) support the argument that increased knowledge on its own does not equate to better decisions or an increase in the use of research evidence. Pardue (1987) and Girot (2000) found that while critical thinking improved with the level of nurses' educational attainment, the frequency of decisions and the perceived difficulty of the decisions themselves were not altered. Lacey (1994) and Rizzuto et al (1994) demonstrate a positive correlation between educational preparation in research methods and utilisation and the use of research in practice. However, the relevance of these studies to the use of evidence-based practice is questionable. Education and training, however, may promote confidence in the use of research material in practice. This is desirable and can have a positive effect on formal research utilisation activity (Funk et al 1995), and consumption of information generally, in the form of health care library use (Wakeham 1996).

Valuing research

A nurse's attitude towards research has been shown to be an important correlate of the use of research-based evidence in decisions (Champion & Leach 1989). Moreover, involvement of nurses as collaborators or data collectors in research activity is a significant predictor of a positive attitude to research generally (Bostrum &

Suter 1983). The extent to which the nurse is involved in the project may have a bearing: inclusion in the analysis or design of research may be more influential in fostering a positive research attitude than limiting involvement to data collection only (Robichaud-Ekstrand & Sherrard 1994).

Valuing change

As well as these factors, individuals hold diverse values around the issue of change per se. For Rogers (1983) people can be classified on a steep 'S' type curve with key points on this curve being the labels of innovator, early adopter, early majority, late majority and laggard. One might assume that having a ward full of innovators would be a positive force for change, but a team needs a balance – the most experienced nurses are often the most cautious and yet are also the most respected by their peers. Respect, clinical credibility and the 'role model' effect are powerful forces in any change strategy.

The overall picture regarding the relationship between variables located within the individual and the use of research-based evidence in decision-making is at best inconclusive, perhaps mirroring the relative lack of impact that individually located variables have on research-based decision-making generally (Varcoe & Hilton 1995). The implications for organisations of these individual factors is that diagnostic work-ups of the likely barriers to change need to incorporate aspects of individual psychology which are difficult to measure and yet may be incredibly powerful. For this reason large-scale 'blitzkrieg' approaches as organisational diagnosis are not likely to succeed. Far better that an organisation concentrates on focused, sensitive, perhaps qualitative diagnoses in defined clinical areas. Such approaches are better able to handle the subtleties of individual factors and provide local contextual information which is rich and able to be used effectively.

Planning for and managing resistance and change

Each of the aforementioned characteristics of complexity is a challenge to nurses' use of research evidence. Lewin's (1951) influential 'force field' theory of resistance to change offers a useful way of conceptualising those forces which might drive and resist evidence-based nursing practice (Figure 9.3). Lewin (1951) also suggests that people need to be 'unfrozen' from their current positions by being

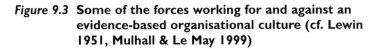

Figure 9.3 Some of the forces working for and against an evidence-based organisational culture (cf. Lewin 1951, Mulhall & Le May 1999)

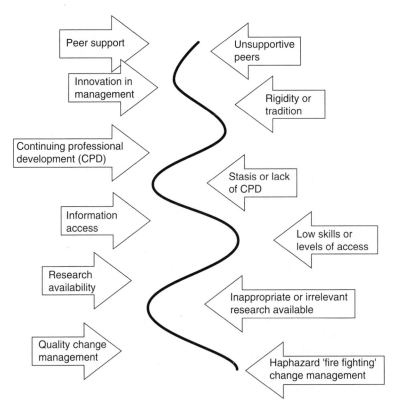

made aware of the need for change. Secondly, the 'force field' needs to be shifted in order to minimise the forces resisting the change. The final stage involves 're-freezing' the change so that it becomes the new status quo and embedded. At this stage you might be asking, 'How should I go about achieving this?'

Two general approaches for changing behaviour are the social marketing model and the precede–proceed model of planned change. It is important to stress that these approaches are theoretical in that they have not been exposed to large-scale evaluation in health care environments. However, what they represent is a way of framing activity and strategy development, and capturing what we do know about changing behaviours in organisations: that diagnosis and planned, multifaceted approaches are likely to yield the best results (Oxman et al 1995).

Social marketing

Social marketing recognises that organisations are made up of relatively homogeneous subgroups and that successful change targets these subgroups. The model has six stages:

1. Research the group(s) you wish to target and identify the resources you have available to help you achieve the change.
2. Select the 'raw materials' for the change you want to introduce. These might include identifying potential change agents, dissemination formats, systems to work through and available skills in the staff. As part of identifying the resources for change it is necessary to break down the staff group into subgroups (as you will be targeting these subgroups for the change). The basis for these subgroups might include factors such as their degree of motivation for change, or confidence with handling research-based information. This stage is also associated with specifying the shape and structure of the strategy involved and the outcomes that one wishes to pursue or avoid.
3. Develop and pilot the materials used to facilitate the change. This will give valuable insight into the likely impact of the materials, their comprehensibility and relevance to the organisation and professional subgroups.
4. Implement the change: this needs careful management and adherence to the time scale for change. Use your knowledge of the subgroups to target materials and employ media creatively to get the messages across.
5. Evaluation: use the outcomes specified in stage 2 as the basis for judging how far the change has progressed and whether or not the groups involved have reached their objectives.
6. Feedback: the results of the intervention are used to strengthen the implementation and refine the change strategy.

Precede–proceed

An alternative to the social marketing approach is the precede–proceed model of change. Its name is derived from the fact that it specifies the steps that should precede any change and the ways in which organisations should proceed with the change (Green et al 1980, Green and Kreuter 1991).

The first stage of the precede–proceed model is concerned with specifying the problem to be addressed and isolating those factors which contribute to the presence of the problem. This stage recognises that problems will have different priorities for different organisational stakeholders and so it is important to try to reach some form of consensus regarding the factors which predispose and contribute to the problem, the importance of these factors and their susceptibility to change. Commonly, this takes the form of a ranking, rating, or 'Delphi' type approach. Common factors include:

- *predisposing*: the perceptions, attitudes, motivations and beliefs of stakeholders involved with the change
- *enabling*: resources such as skills, knowledge (and funds!)
- *reinforcing*: rewards or incentives – even if only in the form of positive feedback.

Having carried out the groundwork, the change is implemented and evaluated with reference to the actual behaviour change observed and the impact it has had on the predisposing, enabling and reinforcing factors.

These are just two of the frameworks available for organisations to draw on and there are many more. Many of these have not been subjected to rigorous empirical testing but they each offer a common set of conditions for 'organising' change. Specifically, they force the manager or clinician considering change to focus on diagnosing the change problem, the antecedents of that problem most amenable to intervention, approaching the implementation of change in a planned and systematic way and evaluating its impact. A good start point for this generic approach to managing change generally is the 'Clinical effectiveness: What's it all about?' resource pack for nurses and health care professionals produced by the NHS Executive (NHS Executive 1999).

An evidence-based toolkit for change?

In the course of our work with nurses we often hear that 'there is nothing out there which tells us what works with changing practice'.

Actually, there is a surprising volume of material that summarises what we know about changing behaviour and which represents the 'state of the art' in terms of managing the transition from abstract research knowledge into improved, and research-informed, professional decisions. The Cochrane Collaboration (http://www. cochrane. co.uk) have an entire systematic review group dedicated to establishing what works in terms of improving professional practice and their output has been summarised in an Effective Health Care Bulletin (NHS CRD 1999), general review articles in journals and policy reports over the past 6 years (Oxman et al 1995).

Developing evidence-based ward literature

The first strategy is not covered by the reviews of existing interventions, but arises out of a general recognition that nurses have limited time available for consulting written sources of information, that many resources are out of date and not evidence-based. Importantly, many sources are poorly organised with few individuals having the ability to rapidly lay their hands on the written information. Moreover, nurses often invest time and considerable amounts of money in compiling these inadequate resources. We suggest that where ward, practice or community teams are committed to maintaining paper-based resources in practice environments, they concentrate on compiling only explicitly evidence-based resources. This strategy will provide a resource which is better suited to clinical decision-making and combats many of the flaws of existing literature- or information-related variables reported earlier in the chapter.

As the NHS embraces electronic information technology (through NHS Net and the National Electronic Library for Health) it is crucial that nurses acquire the skills to handle information effectively. There is no shortcut available to learning the computer and keyboard skills needed to use a personal referencing system or on-line database, but the investment will pay dividends. A first port of call for nurses employed by the NHS or by academic institutions within the UK is the National Electronic Library for Health (NeLH) (http://www.nelh.nhs.uk). This provides an invaluable source of quality-assured information, including links to many of the resources listed in Table 9.1 (accessible under the 'Know how', 'Knowledge' or 'Resources' headings within the electronic library).

Table 9.1 **Sources of evidence-based health care knowledge for a ward or unit library**

Source	Description
Effective Health Bulletins	Based around systematic reviews of effectiveness and cost-effectiveness studies. Produced by the NHS Centre for Reviews and Dissemination (CRD) at the University of York. Dealing with a range of clinical and management topics. Available through National Electronic Library for Health (NeLH) http://www.nelh.nhs.uk and http://www.york.ac.uk
Effectiveness Matters	Complements effective health care, provides updates on the effectiveness of important health interventions for practitioners and decision-makers in the NHS. Covers topics in a shorter more journalistic style, summarising the results of high-quality systematic reviews. Available through NeLH and http://www.york.ac.uk
NHS Centre for Reviews and Dissemination (CRD) Reports	Detailed reports of the systematic reviews carried out by the NHS CRD (in-depth, detailed and comprehensive). Available through NeLH and http://www.york.ac.uk
Evidence-based journals	Journals such as Evidence Based Nursing, Evidence Based Medicine, Evidence Based Mental Health, Evidence Based Healthcare Management, and ACP Journal Club offer concise summaries and clinical commentaries of the best quality research evidence. Evidence Based Nursing available through http://www.evidencebasednursing.com
Epidemiologically based needs assessment	Published by the NHS Executive to support the commissioning process
Health Technology Assessments (HTA)	Some of the NHS HTA programme consists of systematic reviews. Available through NeLH and http://www.hta.nhsweb.nhs.uk
Clinical Evidence	Clinical Evidence is a six monthly, updated compendium of evidence on the effects of common clinical interventions, published by the BMJ Publishing Group. It provides a concise account of the current state of knowledge, ignorance and uncertainty about the prevention and treatment of a wide range of clinical conditions based on thorough searches of the literature. It is not a textbook of medicine nor a book of guidelines. It summarises the best available evidence, and where there is no good evidence, it says so. Available through NeLH and http://www.clinicalevidence.com/

Table 9.1 **(Contd.)**

Source	Description
Cochrane Library	The Cochrane Library contains four databases which can be accessed via the internet (and NHS Net) and local CD-ROM: ■ Cochrane Database of Systematic Reviews: a database of systematic reviews and planned reviews carried out for the Cochrane Collaboration ■ Database of Abstracts of Reviews of Effectiveness (DARE): critically appraised abstracts of systematic reviews. The abstracts are produced by reviewers from the NHS Centre for Reviews and Dissemination at the University of York ■ Cochrane Review Methodology Update: articles, links, and resources for those considering or undertaking a review ■ Cochrane Controlled Trials Register: a register of controlled trials identified by reviewers for the Cochrane Collaboration Available through NeLH and http://www.cochranelibrary.com
National Clinical Guidelines	The Royal College of Nursing is beginning to carry out guidelines (so far in the management of leg ulcers and pain in children). The National Institute for Clinical Excellence is set to produce clinical guidelines based on reviews of good-quality research evidence. At present organisations such as the Scottish Intercollegiate Guidelines Network and the North of England Guidelines Group also produce evidence-based clinical guidelines. Available through NeLH and http://www.rcn.org.uk
MEDLINE and CINAHL	Databases such as MEDLINE and CINAHL are invaluable, especially where the above sources fail to yield relevant information. An internet version of MEDLINE, PubMed, is available through the NeLH and http://www.ncbi.nlm.nih.gov/entrez/query.fcgi

Having diagnosed what the likely environmental barriers are and committed to concentrating efforts on explicitly evidence-based sources, there are other techniques which practitioners should consider in any overall change strategy.

Strategic approaches: breadth versus detail

There are two competing tensions in play in the literature on changing professional behaviour: a high volume of papers dealing exclusively with interventions aimed at changing nursing practice, but using inappropriate methodologies for examining their effectiveness. Conversely, there are studies that use appropriate methods but which do not always focus exclusively on nursing. Moreover, we are faced with a further dichotomy between general and broadly defined strategies: continuing professional development versus the more tightly defined, electronic reminders. Following the spirit of this book, we will focus on those approaches which have been exposed to rigorous empirical scrutiny via systematic reviews.

General approaches

Continuing education

Study days, professional development courses, conference attendance, and post-registration courses are all common features of many nurses' career trajectories and plans. However, the effectiveness of these approaches is far from certain – particularly if divorced from other elements of a change strategy. Five systematic reviews (Beaudry 1989, Bertram and Brooks-Bertram 1977, Davis et al 1995, Lloyd and Abrahamson 1979, Waddell 1991) all examine the impact of educational approaches on changing health care professional behaviours. Waddell (1991) focuses specifically on nurses. The results are contradictory, with most reviews reporting at least some effect but hampered by the poor quality of many of the primary research reports. It is significant, however, that the high-quality systematic reviews (Davis et al 1995) are the ones that conclude that continuing educational approaches are a relatively ineffective way of changing practice. Conversely, those reviews of lesser quality tend towards viewing study days as more effective (Waddell 1991).

Clinical guidelines

Clinical guidelines have proved an influential and attractive mechanism for influencing behaviour in nursing, with the Royal College of Nursing committed to sponsoring, and cooperating in, their production. However, as in the case of continuing professional development, their success should not be assumed uncritically. Thomas et al (1999) have undertaken a systematic review of the role of clinical guidelines as a route to reducing inappropriate variations in practice and promoting the delivery of evidence-based health care (see Chapter 8 for details about the systematic review), and conclude that guidelines as a route to changing practice have only limited utility. They suggest the best advice for nurses wishing to use guidelines to change practice is to learn from the experiences of other groups – notably medicine, and to develop strategies which draw on evidence-based theoretical perspectives (Grol 1992). NHS CRD (1999) found that properly developed guidelines can influence practice, but work best if adapted to local circumstance, used in conjunction with supportive educational strategies and use specific reminders to help professionals in their decision-making.

Of course some strategies, such as integrated care pathways, manage to combine at least some of these elements. Pathways are commonly based around local systems and processes, supported by clinical and managerial teams, based on a guideline format and have reminders built into documentation and monitoring technologies which are often part of larger scale clinical audit. However, we are aware of only limited evidence of their success (Marrie et al 2000) as they have not been exposed to large-scale evaluation.

Other broad approaches

A number of systematic reviews examine the effectiveness of broad dissemination and implementation strategies (Oxman et al 1995; Wensing and Van der Weijden 1998; Yano et al 1995): providing research information alone, management approaches, and social influence approaches. Most of the reviews concur with Oxman and colleagues' (1995) assertion that there are 'no magic bullets' when it comes to changing professional practice or attitudes. Our assessment – based on the evidence – is that multifaceted approaches to change, whilst more expensive, have the most impact. However, this impact is unpredictable and does not always work across each situation.

Specific interventions

A number of systematic reviews examine whether or not specific approaches are useful for clinicians or managers seeking to introduce change. These reviews, or more precisely, the interventions they focus on, can be classified according to the degree of effect on clinical practice: consistently effective, mixed, or little/no impact (Bero et al 1998). Again it should be stressed that in examining these interventions we have valued appropriate evaluative methodology over and above nurse-specific content.

Consistently effective

Educational outreach/detailing

Academic or educational detailing involves trained individuals going out to practice environments to help promote the utilisation of research findings in practice. We have used this approach at York in the area of compression bandaging for venous leg ulceration but it has proved particularly successful in the prescribing arena. Up until now most of the work has been conducted in North American settings with doctors, but the approach may be useful in attempting to change practice amongst nurses in the UK. The effect of outreach approaches is maximised when conducted alongside a social marketing framework. The National Research Register (http://www.update-software.com/NRR/) gives contact details of researchers currently examining the value of educational outreach in the UK and some of these studies are specific to nursing. (For example, 'An evaluation of the effectiveness and cost effectiveness of audit and feedback and educational outreach in improving nursing practice and outcomes', and 'Educational outreach in diabetes to encourage practice nurses to respond to guidelines to control hypertension and hyperlipidaemia in primary and shared care (EDEN): a randomized trial using a blocked reciprocal control design'.) Generally, 'interactive' approaches to educating groups of professionals may yield positive results (Bero et al 1998).

Reminders

Reminders, whether manual or electronic, have been shown to be effective in improving preventative care (Shea et al 1996) and general management of patients. However, it is worth pointing out as nurses increasingly diagnose and treat common conditions (such as asthma), that their effect in relation to improving diagnostic behaviour is uncertain (Hunt et al 1998).

Multifaceted interventions

Combining two or more of audit and feedback, reminders, local consensus processes (see below) and marketing approaches in an overall change strategy offers the highest chance of success (Davis et al 1995, Wensing & Van der Weijden 1998).

Mixed effects

Audit and feedback

It is doubtful that clinical audit, on its own, is a sufficient mechanism for sustained change. Those studies looking at whether audit and feedback approaches to change result in improved behaviours (Balas et al 1996, Buntinx et al 1993, Thomson et al 1999) report at best only moderate effects and see it as less effective than less labour-intensive methods (such as reminders). Audit and feedback, as part of a wider strategy, has some merit; but as a standalone approach to change should not be relied upon.

Local opinion leaders

Thomson et al (1999) report that local opinion leaders as conduits for change have mixed effects on professional practice. However, we do not always know what local opinion leaders do and descriptions of their characteristics are often lacking. Thomson et al (1999) suggest that further research is required to determine the identifying characteristics of leaders and the circumstances in which they are likely to influence the practice of their peers. Bero et al (1998) suggest that colleagues nominated by peers as 'educationally influential' might be a useful characteristic to focus on. Our own work, however, suggests that it is 'clinical credibility' (in the form of experience) rather than research competence or awareness which proves influential in getting nurses to engage with imparted information (Thompson et al 2000). In this multiple-case site study, we found that nurses often perceived other nurses as an influential block on them using research. Local opinion leaders (often those embodying the clinical nurse specialist role) were a powerful force for change.

Local consensus approaches

Mulhall & Le May (1999, page 200) recognise that 'ownership of the [change] project by nurses is important' and this statement is borne out by the evidence. Bero et al (1998) report that inclusion of stakeholder professionals in discussions to ensure their perception of the change problem as 'important' is developed and their response defined as 'appropriate' can exert some effect. However, the results of their scrutiny are mixed and consensus alone should not be relied upon.

Patient-mediated interventions
If a patient asked you to justify your choice of wound dressing or urinary catheter would it change your approach? This kind of question lies at the core of patient-mediated interventions. By providing information to patients to use in a specific way in professional consultations they can, in theory, exert an impact on the behaviour of clinicians. For example, many professionals are increasingly encountering the 'internet informed' patient and anecdotally both of us have encountered health care professionals who claim that this 'makes them think twice' about the sorts of information and care provided. However, here too results are mixed and patient-mediated approaches are not a sufficient standalone mechanism for cultural shift.

Little or no effect

Worryingly, those sources of research-based knowledge which many nurses rely on, such as didactic lecture-style study days, passively disseminated clinical practice guidelines, lecture notes, educational videos and protocols, seem to exert the least (if any) effect on professional practice. Freemantle et al (1999) in a review of printed educational materials found no statistically significant improvements in practice. Similarly, Bero and colleagues (1998) report that didactic-style educational meetings are not a useful route for inducing change in practice.

Real life examples of changing practice and culture

The following three examples provide mini vignettes of the complexities associated with influencing culture. Case studies 9.1 and 9.2 come from the King's Fund Report 'Getting better with evidence' (Wye & McClenahan 2000) and case study 9.3 from some on-going work which one of the author's (ML) contributed to in relation to performance indication and quality in the NHS.

Case study 9.1: A nurse-led anticoagulation clinic

A group of secondary care Trusts were targeted by the local health authority as suitable for the establishment of nurse-led anticoagulation clinics. Their strategy focused on using a combination of clinical guidelines, training and local opinion leaders to influence the approach. Guidelines were drawn up by consultant haematologists for nurses in conjunction with safety objectives and a short two-page protocol for the management of deep vein thrombosis and pulmonary embolism. To complement this, two nurses were given intensive (14 sessions in the first 3 months) and personalised training by two consultants. The two nurses also visited well-established nurse-led clinics in other areas. The overall leadership and 'steer' for the project was provided by the two respected and enthusiastic medical consultants. The project was audited every 3 months and the results fed back into the service planning and implementation loop. Data collected were a combination of clinical outcomes (such as mortality in stroke inpatients) and more qualitative end-user (patient and doctor) views on the service. The service also utilised a form of paper reminder in the form of a questionnaire on atrial fibrillation sent to local GPs which acted to reinforce the presence of the service.

The service is now well-established in two main sites and being developed in a third. Numbers of patients on warfarin have increased and the general feeling is that nurses run the clinics well and that as a model of service delivery the framework is successful and sustainable. However, the project did have to contend with funding and IT problems. Despite the perceived success of the project, the outcomes audit reveals that admissions for strokes have not fallen from the 212 and 198 per year established at baseline in each site. The authors are at a loss to explain this but it does highlight the issue that perceived improvements in a service may not be accompanied by a change in patient outcomes. Change is often long term and measures of 'success' multidimensional and sensitive – because of this reason it may be advantageous to examine 'softer' indicators of success such as the levels of satisfaction with the process of care delivery.

Case study 9.2: Primary care leg ulcer clinics

A group of tissue viability specialist nurses (TVNs) working in an inner-city area wanted to develop, implement and audit their local guidelines on managing leg ulcers and then set up two community-based leg ulcer clinics. The aim of this was to reduce variations in practice and outcomes across the Trust and to reduce inappropriate referrals to an already busy complex wound clinic.

The nurses' developed a fivefold strategy:

1. Locally developed guidelines: These were based on an inclusive, multidisciplinary, development process which was actively 'marketed' in

Trust settings at lunchtimes.

2. Opinion leaders: The two well-respected TVNs worked with nurses on a part-time basis and ensured that they also worked with consultants and local GPs.

3. Educational workshops: These took place 'in-service' and were aimed at familiarising nurses with the guidelines, but crucially, learning to relate the guidelines to real patients and patient problems.

4. Targeted meetings and multidisciplinary training: These focused on generating sufficient interest in practitioners so that they wanted to host clinics. Moreover, these involved targeting the most enthusiastic practitioner in a local team in order that they would persuade their – more sceptical – colleagues.

5. Training and feedback: The TVN visited each clinic once a month and offered real time training, support and, crucially, the application of the guidelines during patient consultations.

This approach has led to the development of two clinics with a third in progress with broad cross-disciplinary support for the new ways of working. However, the team failed to collect patient data before or after the development of the clinics which meant they had no baseline criteria for measuring their success. As well as this design fault, the team had to struggle against the very real constraints of underfunding, recruitment difficulties, competing priorities and variable morale and enthusiasm amongst staff. The qualitative comments of staff, in particular, reveal that relatively small changes such as changing the ways in which clinical nurse specialists work (giving them a Trust-wide remit with responsibility for individual training and professional development) can yield good results – even in the context of a far from perfect strategy:

> Having (the clinical nurse specialist) there to discuss different things makes a difference. When you are seeing seven leg ulcers in a row, it leads to better practice. We are using the leg ulcer care program lots ... the professional development is the best part of it. (Wye & McClenahan 2000, page 36)

So a relatively small change can have a significant impact on the development of others' expertise and professional development. Importantly, the team involved learned from their mistakes and were trying to factor in the solutions for the future:

> We would invest a proportion of the project's resources in a baseline audit because demonstrating improvement in healing rates provides the ultimate

proof that an initiative to upgrade the care of patients with leg ulcers is working. (Wye & McClenahan 2000, page 36)

Ultimately, the researchers conclude that the team's greatest (cultural) achievement was their contribution to the replacement of 'a severely fragmented, demoralized organization with one where staff are enthusiastic and open to learning'.

Case study 9.3: Accessing guidance for best practice on-line

As we said right at the beginning of this chapter, 'managing culture' is not straightforward; attempts to do so can have unpredictable and dysfunctional effects. Thus, whilst everyone would agree that a culture of excellence is desirable, trying to get there may have the reverse effect. The example below is part of an interview conducted by ML with a Trust chief executive who was talking about the recent introduction of a ward-based system for accessing guidance about best practice on-line.

> But of course what we'll do is – cos it's computerized – we know who's accessing it where and when; and if we keep an eye on that and if we find that pockets of areas aren't using it well then we'll kind of target them for sort of well you know – why aren't you using it? Is it because you don't like using it? Is it because you aren't interested in kind of the right things to do, or what? And not in a sort of big brother sort of way but in an encouraging facilitative sort of way and encourage its use.

That he was expecting resistance to 'best practice' is pretty clear – although he is apparently mystified by why people might resist. He is also aware that his attempts to create an evidence-based culture run the risk of creating a 'Big Brother is watching you' sort of culture rather than the desired one.

This last (very brief) example is here as a form of caveat for those considering trying to change organisational culture. Even with diagnosis, a theoretical framework, a multiapproach strategy using validated techniques, the results are often far from certain and nothing can be assumed.

Conclusion: culture, practice change and evidence-based health care

This chapter has shown how complex an entity organisational culture is and how difficult it is to try to mould something that is, by definition, malleable and contingent on so many other factors. Never the less, we have outlined a number of strategies, which, if used in conjunction with broad and specific interventions, could reasonably be expected to yield some results.

Most people would agree that evidence-based health care should be a reality but very often tips on how to deliver the necessary behavioural (and by implication cultural) changes are lacking. This chapter has argued that strategy and working with proven approaches can help add the local detail necessary to complement the national directives.

As Oxman et al (1995) point out, there are 'no magic bullets' when attempting organisational change. However, by strategically arming oneself with a number of different techniques for changing culture and behaviour, you can at least give yourself and your team a fighting chance of successfully introducing change. To conclude then, the clinician or manager considering change should employ a good diagnostic work-up of the factors likely to impinge or promote research use in decisions. This diagnostic work-up should focus on the levels of individuals, teams and the organisation. Clinicians seeking change should consider strategically targeting barriers and subgroups at each of these levels. Moreover, initial efforts should focus on those areas over which the team has a modicum of control (for example, the text-based ward resources amassed by the ward, unit or practice; the roles of key individuals such as the clinical nurse specialist or the link nurse role; or the support and nature of skills training). Be aware of the likely time scale involved and the non-linear progress of change. Ensure the process is cyclical, with audit and with feedback 'built in'.

Summary

- Evidence-based change is a national policy imperative and unavoidable in practice.
- Evidence-based culture is one which is totally committed to balanced decisions that give due weight to research evidence, patient preference, available resources and clinical expertise. This commitment is manifest at the level of the individual, clinical teams and health care systems.

- Successful strategies for change are likely to be multifaceted, targeted at specific cultural groups in the organisation.
- Specific groups for targeted and planned change interventions are best identified through sensitive diagnostic strategies.
- Common barriers to change amongst nurses often relate to the information they have available, professional cultural resistance to some forms of evidence, environmental factors, such as the availability of evidence, and individual psychology relating to change.
- Theoretical models of and for change, such as social marketing, may prove useful as a way of structuring change strategies, but evidence to date is lacking.
- Consistently effective interventions include educational outreach, electronic or paper-based reminders and multifacted approaches.
- Audit and feedback alone has a mixed and unpredictable impact on changing professional behaviour and culture.
- Didactic study days, clinical guidelines and protocols which are passively disseminated have little or no effect on practice.

References

Balas EA, Austin SM, Mitchell J et al 1996 The clinical value of computerized information services: a review of 98 randomized clinical trials. Archives of Family Medicine 5: 271–278

Beaudry JS 1989 The effectiveness of continuing medical education: a quantitative synthesis. Journal of Continuing Education for Health Professionals 9: 285–307

Bero LA, Grilli R, Grimshaw JM et al 1998 Closing the gap between research and practice: an overview of systematic reviews of interventions to promote the implementation of research findings. British Medical Journal 317: 465–468

Bertram DA, Brooks-Bertram PA 1977 The evaluation of continuing medical education: a literature review. Health Education Monographs 5: 330–362

Bostrum J, Suter WN 1993 Research utilization: making the link to practice. Journal of Nursing Staff Development 9(1): 28–34

Brown SJ 1999 Knowledge for health care practice: a guide to using research evidence. London: WB Saunders

Buntinx F, Winkens R, Grol R et al 1993 Influencing diagnostic and preventative performance in ambulatory care by feedback and reminders. A review. Family Practice 10: 219–228

Calas MB, Smircich L 1987 Organizational culture: a critical assessment. In: Jablin FM, Putnam LL, Roberts KH et al (eds) Handbook of organizational communication. Beverly Hills: Sage

Cameron G, Wren AM 1999 Reconstructing organizational culture: a process using multiple perspectives. Public Health Nursing 16(2): 96–101

Champion VL, Leach A 1989 Variables related to research utilisation in nursing: an empirical investigation. Journal of Advanced Nursing 14: 705–710

Coyle LA, Sokow AG 1990 Innovation adoption behavior among nurses. Nursing Research 39: 176–180

Crow R, Chase J, Lamond D 1995 The cognitive component of nursing assessment: an analysis. Journal of Advanced Nursing 22: 206–212

Davies HTO, Nutley SM, Mannion R 2000 Organizational culture and quality of health care. Quality in Health Care 9: 111–119

Davis DA, Thomson MA, Oxman AD et al 1995 Changing physician performance: a systematic review of the effect of continuing medical education strategies. Journal of the American Medical Association 274: 700–705

Department of Health 1998 A first class service. London: The Stationery Office

DiCenso A, Cullum N, Ciliska D 1998 Implementation forum. Implementing evidence-based nursing: some misconceptions. Evidence Based Nursing 1(2): 38–40

Dunn V, Crighton N, Williams K, Row B, Seers K 1998 Using research for practice: a UK experience of the BARRIERS Scale. Journal of Advanced Nursing 27: 1203–1210

Freemantle N, Harvey EL, Wolf F, Grimshaw JM, Grilli R, Bero LA 1999 Printed educational materials to improve the behavior of health care professionals and patient outcomes (Cochrane Review). In: The Cochrane Library, Disk Issue 1. Oxford: Update Software

Funk S, Champagne MT, Wiese RA, Tornquist EM 1991 Barriers: the barriers to research utilization scale. Applied Nursing Research 4(1): 39–45

Funk SG, Tornquist EM, Champagne MT 1995 Barriers and facilitators of research utilization. Nursing Clinics of North America 30(3): 395–407

Gabriel Y 1999 Organizations in depth. Sage: London

Girot EA 2000 Graduate nurses: critical thinkers or better decision makers? Journal of Advanced Nursing 31(2): 288–297

Green LW, Kreuter M 1991 Health promotion planning: an educational and environmental approach. London: Mayfield Publishing

Green LW, Kreuter MW, Deeds SG et al 1980 Health education planning: a diagnostic approach. California: Mayfield Publishing

Grol R 1992 Implementing guidelines in general practice care. Quality Health Care 1: 184–191

Hunt DL, Haynes RB, Hanna SE et al 1998 Effects of computer based decision support on physician performance and patient outcomes. A systematic review. Journal of the American Medical Association 280: 1339–1346

Jacavone J, Dostal M 1992 A descriptive study of nursing judgement in the assessment and management of cardiac pain. Advances in Nursing Science 15: 54–63

Lacey EA 1994 Research utilization in nursing practice – a pilot study. Journal of Advanced Nursing 19: 987–995

Lewin K 1951 Field theory and learning. In: Cartwright D (ed) Field theory in social science: select theoretical papers. New York: Harper Collins

Lloyd JS, Abrahamson S 1979 Effectiveness of continuing medical education: a review of the evidence. Evaluation in the Health Professions 2: 251–280

Marrie TJ, Lau CY, Wheeler SL, Wong CJ, Vandervoort MK, Feagan BG 2000 A controlled trial of a critical pathway for treatment of community-acquired pneumonia. Journal of the American Medical Association 283(6): 749–755

Muir Gray JA 1997 Evidence-based healthcare: how to make health policy and management decisions. Edinburgh: Churchill Livingstone

Mulhall A, Le May A 1999 Nursing research: dissemination and implementation. London: Churchill Livingstone

NHS CRD (NHS Centre for Reviews and Dissemination) 1999 Getting evidence into practice. Effective Health Care Bulletin 5(1)

NHS Executive 1999 Clinical effectiveness: what it's all about. http://www.doh. gov.uk/pub/docs/doh/aep.pdf

Nilson Kajermo K, Nordstrom G, Krusebrant A, Bjorvell A 1998 Barriers to and facilitators of research utilisation, as perceived by a group of registered nurses in Sweden. Journal of Advanced Nursing 27: 798–807

Nilson Kajermo K, Nordstrom G, Krusebrant A, Bjorvell H 2000 Perceptions of research utilization: comparisons between healthcare professionals, nursing students and a reference group of nurse clinicians. Journal of Advanced Nursing 31(1): 99–109

Oxman A, Thomson MA, Davis DA, Haynes RB 1995 No magic bullets: a systematic review of 102 trials of interventions to improve professional practice. Canadian Medical Association Journal 153(10): 1423–1431

Parahoo K 2000 Barriers to, and facilitators of, research utilisation among nurses in Northern Ireland. Journal of Advanced Nursing 31(1): 89–98

Pardue SF 1987 Decision making skills and critical thinking ability among associate degree, diploma, baccalaureate, and master's prepared nurses. Journal of Nursing Education 26: 354–361

Parker M 2000 Organizational culture and identity: unity and division at work. Sage: London

Retsas A 2000 Barriers to using research evidence in nursing practice. Journal of Advanced Nursing 31(3): 599–606

Rizzuto C, Bostrum, Suter WN, Cheniotz WC 1994 Predictors of nurses' involvement in research activities. Western Journal of Nursing Research 16: 193–204

Robichaud-Ekstrand S, Sherrard H 1994 Cardiac nurses' perceptions of nursing research. Progress in Cardiovascular Issues 9(3): 7–15

Rogers E 1993 Diffusion of innovations. New York: Free Press

Sackett DL, Strauss SE, Richardson WS, Rosenberg W, Haynes RB 2000 Evidence based medicine: how to practice and teach EBM. London: Churchill Livingstone

Schon D 1983 The reflective practitioner: how professionals think in action. New York: Basic Books

Secretary of State for Health 1998 A first class service: quality in the new NHS. London: Department of Health

Secretary of State for Health 2000 The NHS plan. London: Department of Health

Shea S, DuMouchel W, Bahamonde L 1996 A meta-analysis of 16 randomized controlled trials to evaluate computer-based clinical reminder systems for preventative care in the ambulatory setting. Journal of the American Medical Information Association 3: 399–409

Thomas L, Cullum N, McColl E, Rousseau N, Soutter J, Steen N 1999 Clinical guidelines in nursing, midwifery and other professions allied to medicine (Cochrane Review). In: The Cochrane Library, Disk Issue 1. Oxford: Update Software

Thompson C, McCaughan D, Cullum N, Sheldon TA, Thompson DR, Mulhall A 2000 Nurses' use of research information in clinical decision making: a descriptive and analytical study – final report. London: NHS R&D, NCC SDO

Thomson MA, Oxman AD, Davis DA, Haynes RB, Freemantle N, Harvey EL 1999 Outreach visits to improve health professional practice and health care outcomes (Cochrane Review). In: The Cochrane Library, Disk Issue 1. Oxford: Update Software

Varcoe C, Hilton A 1995 Factors affecting acute-nurses' use of research findings. Canadian Journal of Nursing Research 27(4): 51–71

Waddell DL 1991 The effects of continuing education on nursing practice: a meta-analysis. Journal of Continuing Education in Nursing 22: 113–118

Wakeham M 1996 What nurses think of library services: a research study. Nursing Standard 10(28): 40–43

Wensing M, Van der Weijden TRG 1998 Implementing guidelines and innovations in general practice: which interventions are effective. British Journal of General Practice 48: 991–997

White JE, Natisio DG, Kobert SN, Engberg SJ 1992 Content and process in clinical decision making by nurse practitioners. Image: Journal of Nursing Scholarship 24(2): 153–158

Wye L, McClenahan J 2000 Getting better with evidence: Experiences of putting evidence into practice. London: King's Fund

Yano EM, Fink A, Hirsch SH et al 1995 Helping practices reach primary care goals. Lessons from the literature. Archives of Internal Medicine 155: 1146–1156

10

Implementing best evidence in clinical practice

Lin Perry

Key points

- Where to start?
  - Identifying appropriate topics to address
  - Choosing a project manager
  - Diagnosing the situation
- What changes are needed?
  - Ensuring change is based on best available evidence
  - Turning evidence into recommendations
  - Establishing key objectives
- How to implement the changes
  - Developing a dissemination and implementation strategy
  - General approaches to managing change
  - Specific approaches to managing change
- Evaluating the progress and effects of the changes.

Introduction

The aim of this chapter is to help nurses understand how the implementation of best evidence can be applied in everyday practice. It draws on ground covered in previous chapters and presents information in the context of real clinical settings. Examples are taken extensively, although not exclusively, from the South Thames Evidence-based Practice Project (STEP), a series of nine projects run concurrently across the old South Thames region of England within a framework of outside evaluation by King's College between 1997 and 2000.

Background to the STEP project

STEP was funded by a regional Research and Development Directorate within the Department of Health. The aim was to implement and evaluate evidence-based practice. Eight topics were identified, representing areas of practice supported by relatively better-developed evidence bases (nutrition (two projects) and rehabilitation in acute stroke, discharge-planning, leg ulcer management, pressure damage prevention, promotion of breast feeding, continence care and family intervention for schizophrenia). A common framework was established incorporating the development and implementation of evidence-based guidelines, preceded and followed by audit of clinical practice and patient outcomes. Trusts within the region were invited to participate. A total of nine were chosen and collaborative partnerships were set up with four university departments.

Project managers/co-ordinators were jointly appointed with eight out of the nine coming from outside the host Trusts. Although not a specific requirement, six were nursing appointments, with one dietician, a midwife and a medical social worker. The individual projects were accomplished within 3 years. This included the external evaluation of processes and outcomes across the nine sites.

This chapter draws in detail on one of the projects undertaken in a 700-bed district general hospital of an acute Trust in a large South London borough. In common with many Trusts, the hospital had a stroke rehabilitation ward where approximately one-third of stroke patients were located for part of their stay with the remainder spent, with other stroke patients, in predominantly medical and care-of-the-elderly wards. The project aimed to develop, implement and evaluate the impact of evidence-based guidelines for nutritional support of patients with acute stroke throughout the hospital. To achieve this a nurse project manager (from a clinical–academic background) was appointed to lead a multiprofessional group comprising lead stroke clinicians, managers of the Trust and a university professor; patient-representation was sought and achieved indirectly. This group was responsible for developing the guidelines and a local dissemination and implementation strategy. The major topics of the guidelines were screening and assessment of swallowing; other stroke-related eating difficulties and nutritional risk; management of nutritional compromise and eating impairments such as dysphagia, lack of postural control and arm movement, communication, visual, perceptual and cognitive deficits. Evaluation was achieved through a combination of analysis of documentation from relevant professional groups, interview and questionnaires with staff, assessments and interviews with patients and carers, observation of ward meal-time events.

How is this relevant to me?

Experiences gained from this and the other STEP projects will have direct relevance for practitioners and clinical governance leads charged with implementing evidence-based changes in practice. The diversity of project topics, settings (encompassing an accident and emergency department, acute and rehabilitation wards, outpatient and day centres, general practice and domiciliary locations) and participants produced a wealth of information about what worked in which contexts. For those embarking upon or contemplating changing health care practice it will offer an illustrated 'basic steps' approach. It will supply examples and explanations for what worked and what did not work, allowing readers to make comparisons with their own environments and identify directly relevant information.

Where to start?

Identifying appropriate topics to address

Many topics arise directly from nurses' everyday practice as problems in need of solution or questions to be answered. For individual nurses, the process of finding best evidence is becoming easier. For example, the National Electronic Library for Health (NeLH) (at www.nelh.nhs.uk) offers search facilities for a number of sites of high-quality evidence such as the Clinical Evidence journal, the Cochrane Library, TRIP and SUMSearch. From these, the nurse may find an answer to the problem and may be able to enact it without resource considerations or impacting colleagues' practice. However, in most instances other practitioners are also involved. Even when choosing the most appropriate dressing for a specific wound there are wider considerations: if the evidence indicates dressing A, is it available? If not, why not? If it is, but the dressing is later removed and the patient re-presents, will colleagues also apply knowledge of wound care research in choosing a replacement? Hence individual nurses usually need to think more broadly and beyond their own practice in pursuit of best outcomes for their patients.

In this situation, changing practice will require energy, motivation and support from others which will need to be sustained over a period of time; careful selection of the topic is therefore important. There are several key considerations. Patient benefit is of first importance. The primary aim of evidence-based practice has been defined as identification and application of 'the most efficacious interventions to maximise the quality and quantity of life for individual patients' (Sackett et al 1997, page 4); benefiting patients could therefore be considered an intrinsic feature. However, it is sometimes not enough that the literature identifies benefits for patients; clinicians have to be persuaded that these will accrue for their patients and be worth the time and trouble that changing working practices entails. The persuasion (and change management) process may not be easy and will make considerable demands upon the person driving or responsible for the changes.

Hence, personal involvement, engagement and motivation to pursue the topic are prerequisites when choosing a topic. If change leaders cannot sustain enthusiastic belief in the merits of changing practice this is unlikely to be engendered in practitioners. Evaluating nine projects, Redfern et al (2000, page iv) describe the project leaders requiring 'motivation and energy to persevere when the going gets tough and obstacles seem to be insurmountable'. Doherty et al (2000, page 15) and Miller et al (1999) highlight the considerable time and emotional investment entailed in steering projects to successful completion. From the outset the motivation and energy of those driving the change are essential. Next, it is sensible to think about how this may be recruited from others.

Consider local and national views on the topic

What are the opinions of patients, colleagues, clinicians and managers? It was apparent for one of the STEP projects that patients with stroke were dissatisfied with current practices, reflected in letters of complaint both locally and nationally (ACHCEW 1997). Internal satisfaction surveys or clinical audits may also provide a useful source of information; prior to commencement of the STEP nutrition in stroke project, local Community Health Council audits had flagged nutrition in hospital as a local issue, enhancing its priority for managers (Perry et al 2000). Managerial attention may be focused where a topic addresses regional and national priorities. For example, nutritional support for stroke patients

- addresses a national research priority (stroke, Department of Health 2000a)
- features in the patient-focused benchmark for food and nutrition (Department of Health 2001a) and the National Clinical Guidelines for stroke (Intercollegiate Working Party 2000)
- is encompassed within the National Service Framework for Older People (Department of Health 2001b).

Considering factors influencing change, Upton & Brooks (1995) employ a 'change equation' (of f $(D, V, S) > R$), anticipating success where the combination of dissatisfaction (D) with the present situation, a vision (V) of a more desirable future and knowledge of the first steps (S) required to achieve this combine to exceed resistance (R) to or cost of change. Within the STEP stroke project, there was general dissatisfaction with dysphagia management combined with nursing and therapists' aspirations towards a more streamlined, faster process but with specific concerns expressed by individual clinicians. Once the dissatisfaction, vision and resistances were recognised and first steps agreed (i.e. methods for speeding screening and referral without over-riding decision-making processes), changes took place (Perry et al 2000).

The evidence

Any change in practice requires commitment from practitioners and managers. There may be training, cost and time implications, and there is often a need to reassess current methods of working. It is therefore important to consider how best to present the project so as to gain support. What evidence is there to defend a course of action other than the status quo? How good is it? In setting out to persuade clinicians to alter their behaviour, both the quantity and especially the quality of evidence are important. Respected international and national institutions conduct systematic reviews of research evidence and/or present guidance for a wide range of topics (e.g. the Cochrane

Library, the National Institute of Clinical Excellence and the NHS Centre for Reviews and Dissemination and the Scottish Intercollegiate Guidelines Network (SIGN) and a relevant report may be available. However, in many areas evidence is limited. For example, national evidence-based guidelines for rehabilitation interventions after acute stroke comprise 60 recommendations, of which 24 are grade A (defined here as being derived from meta-analysis of randomised controlled trials (RCTs) or at least one RCT), 16 are grade B (based on at least one well-designed controlled, quasi-experimental or descriptive study) and 20 are grade C (reliant upon expert committee report, opinions and/or experience of respected authorities) (Intercollegiate Working Party 2000).

Altogether one-third of rehabilitation topics in the guideline are not supported by any evidence other than published expert clinical opinion. This is no denigration of clinical expertise; in many instances it represents 'best available evidence'. However where the opinions of local experts are not in tune with published recommendations of 'respected authorities' the latter may not be sufficient to effect changes in practice in the face of other competing resistance factors and the prevailing norms of peer group behaviour (Clinical Standards Advisory Group 1998). This may not deter practitioners from addressing a topic which has strong local support. However gaining support for changes underpinned by grade C evidence which local 'experts' do not endorse is likely to present considerable challenge. The practicalities of ensuring changes are based on best available evidence are considered in more detail in the sections on Finding the evidence and Appraising the evidence (pages 257 and 258).

Summary

Altogether, there are a number of factors to consider when thinking about pursuing evidence-based practice development in a given topic.

- Ensure personal engagement with the issue; motivation and energy are crucial.
- Opt for topics which address local priorities and concerns, to maximise local support.
- Identify links with key policy objectives and national strategies to enlist high-level backing.
- Involve/reflect users' views to ensure relevance to their needs.

■ Consider the strength of evidence on the subject; rigorously developed guidance or evidence from well-conducted systematic reviews are likely to be more persuasive than consensus statements.

First steps

Choosing a project manager

A primary consideration is the practice development or project manager/co-ordinator role – the person who will hold day-to-day responsibility. Having the right person with the right skills located in the right post within the organisation has been repeatedly identified as crucial for clinical effectiveness/practice development work (Miller et al 1999, Redfern et al 2000, page 155). Miller et al (1999) stress matching the actual post with changes planned; ensuring adequate positional and legitimate authority with salary scale reflecting skills and level of responsibility.

The range of skills required by the STEP project managers spanned communication, research and audit skills, clinical credibility, guideline development and change management experience (Ross & McLaren 2000, page 25). Even more essential was the ability to learn fast and crest steep learning curves. None met all criteria at appointment. The nurse who occupies the position may have worked locally for many years and be well acquainted not just with the workplace teams or surroundings but with the whole institution and local health care provision. However, practice development initiatives are also feasible and appropriate when initiated by a nurse new to the area; strengths and limitations attach to both positions.

'Insider' status carries obvious immediate advantages; the nurse knows the system, and knows who does what and who to persuade to make things happen. Access to data, personnel and clinical areas may be automatic, and clinical credibility with staff has already been established. However, because the nurse is well known, making a role transition/presenting themselves in a different light may not be straightforward. Doherty et al (2000, pages 14–15) describe difficulties and workload pressures when staff and managers continued to perceive an individual as a clinical nurse specialist despite a role change to practice development. Objectivity for organisational analysis and observation of working practices entails extra effort to see past the familiar. This also presents potential for bias where the nurse may be evaluating practice of which they were a key player, and which represents considerable past personal investment. This situation may also pose personal difficulties if colleagues and friends construe evaluation as criticism.

The position of the 'incomer' is the reverse of this. Neither is better; both require awareness of potential problems and ability to capitalise on strengths. Irrespective of the post holder's insider/incomer status, they should be appointed early enough to contribute to project planning (Redfern et al 2000, pages 141 and 166) and to allow time to mentally step out of the immediate situation and establish the broader picture, referred to as a 'diagnostic analysis' (NHS CRD 1999). They should resist the impatience and desire to start making changes immediately; time invested at this point repays with interest later.

Diagnosing the situation

The organisational environment

A key consideration is the current macro organisational context. Of the nine Trusts involved in the STEP projects three underwent major reorganisation or merger within the life of the projects, two within the first 6 months. One project manager describes a period during which 'everyone senior was either fearful for their jobs, applying for others or settling into new ones . . . a tense and competitive atmosphere for months' (Bignell, personal communication). Redfern et al (2000, page 155) describe this as 'particularly disruptive . . . (especially) when changes occurred during the early stages of the project'. Trust mergers, restructuring and service reconfiguration are not uncommon but a time of organisational change may not be good timing to seek support for changes in practice; at the very least, practice changes must be planned to take other changes into account (Bignell et al 2000, pages 9–10).

Even where organisations were not currently involved in major restructuring, effects of recent changes were felt by staff in many Trusts, e.g. where closure of a neighbouring accident and emergency department accrued workload changes; where wards/departments had relocated or therapy teams had been reconfigured. Many staff reported a sense of 'change-overload' and expressed low tolerance of more change (Doherty et al 2000, page 14). However, it is worth bearing in mind that perceptions of change may vary according to management and presentation. Examples were given where changes to the same workplace perceived as ordered from above with little consultation resulted in stress and resentment, but where consensual reorganisation was seen as mutually beneficial for staff and patients.

Next take a close look at the organisation's priorities, structures and strategic plans. There are a variety of ways of achieving this; for example, reviewing public reports, human resources information, clinical audits, minutes of key group meetings (e.g. of Trust Board, departmental heads, charge nurses); observation of meetings; interviews, focus groups, informal discussions with key figures (Ross & McLaren 2000, pages 32–33). If the selected topic fits within an identified priority area, high-level support may be easier to recruit. Explore existing routes of information dissemination, education and training, avenues by which changes may be introduced. The better the 'fit' between the change initiative and existing priorities and structures, the less time and effort required to introduce it and perhaps greater likelihood of success (Miller et al 1999).

Stakeholders and practitioner opinion leaders

The next stage involves identifying the key players in the topic and for the project, including service users and stakeholders (those with a vested interest in the issue). All groups who may be affected by the proposed changes should be represented by appropriate practitioners, and involved in discussions from the outset. A group representative may be the head of department, someone with recognised expertise in a specific area, for example a senior neurophysio to represent physiotherapy in a stroke project, or a local opinion leader such as the ward sister or an enthusiastic staff nurse. In one of the STEP projects, nomination of a dynamic F-grade staff nurse resulted in her being one of the first to complete training and incorporate dysphagia screening within her daily practice; subsequently her ward demonstrated fastest and most complete uptake of the new role (Perry et al 2000).

The views of stakeholders and opinion leaders to the topic and the changes that are envisaged should be explored. Relationships between individuals' beliefs, attitudes, intentions and behaviours are seldom direct and straightforward. However, whilst poor predictors, attitudes clearly influence behaviour. In discussion with key individuals in advance of a project focused on nutrition support post stroke, it became clear that the risk of inappropriate treatment was a major concern (Perry et al 2000). Decisions about nutritional support for severely disabled patients who are perceived to have poor prognoses can be ethically difficult. Artificial nutritional support is regarded as treatment; whilst provision of 'normal' food and fluid is a human right, clinicians are not obliged to provide treatment believed to be futile (BMA 1999). However, prognostication in acute stroke is an inexact science and the problems of prediction can be compounded by differences of interpretation where future quality of life is the issue. One method of addressing these uncertainties, preferred by some practitioners, was to 'wait and see'; to maintain hydration but withhold nutrition, sometimes through a protracted period of uncertainty. Exploring the origins of this approach revealed isolated incidents, sometimes decades earlier, the emotional effects of which were still felt. In this instance without appreciation of underpinning attitudes it might have been difficult to understand behaviour.

A whole raft of issues may need to be considered when making judgements about the focus of project activities. O'Tuathail et al (2000, page 27) implemented standardised multidisciplinary assessment for older people prior to discharge based on a set of assessment measures assembled via professional consensus (Royal College of Physicians/British Geriatrics Society 1992). It was found that a key individual had reservations about one component; universal screening for depression. It was felt that the tool for screening might not transfer from a research setting to everyday clinical practice; it would be oversensitive and identify clinical depression where patients were experiencing distress accompanying ill-health and removal from their home environment. Unnecessary medication and iatrogenic morbidity would incur; time requirements for comprehensive screening in hospital were unrealistic and sudden increases in patients discharged with diagnoses of depression would overwhelm community resources. It was foreseen that unnecessary additional workload would distract attention from those really in need, who were believed to be satisfactorily but intuitively identified as a function of clinical expertise. Eventually a compromise position was agreed allowing formal screening by senior nursing staff whenever suspicion of depression was roused.

It is useful to identify a link person with senior Trust management. This is usually someone with managerial responsibilities who can communicate and connect Trust and project aims and strategies, including resource issues. Redfern et al (2000, page 155) discuss the importance of this post and suggest the optimal choice is someone senior enough to have authority to make decisions and mobilise responses speedily but also junior enough to have time for the project and closeness/more intimate knowledge of the clinical environment. Their attitude towards the project is also important. A clinical lead described as anxious and ambivalent was believed to have conveyed mixed messages about the project to staff. On evaluation, this project was 'not effective' in influencing global staff outcomes (attitudes and perceptions) although patients' health status benefited. These findings may indicate insensitivity of measurement tools in this environment (Redfern et al 2000, page 140); they may also reflect the effect of mixed messages from a very influential manager.

Grassroots workers

Similar considerations argue for investigation of views of grassroots staff. These are the people who will be asked to enact new ways of working, who will be expected to change their work patterns or activities. One of the key areas to explore includes the priority they accord the topic. Redfern et al note that practitioners in all projects and disciplines reported staff shortages and heavy workloads (2000, page 49); in such circumstances prioritisation of activities is inevitable. The low status accorded some project activities is believed to have hampered guideline implementation, e.g. continence (Bignell et al 2000, pages 20 and 27), leg ulcer care (Doherty et al 2000, page 13), nutrition (Love et al 2000, page 28). It may be necessary to spend time presenting information highlighting the importance and relevance of the topic to all health care practitioners, or to ask project team members to address this within their professional groups.

It is also worth exploring the anticipated impact of the practice change upon workload patterns. Doherty et al (2000, page 14) describe a vicious circle in which lack of time to release community staff nurses for training in leg ulcer management had resulted in a habit of referral to the specialist leg ulcer team. Specialist care effectively decreased community team workload, so there was no motivation to release staff for training which would lighten the load on the specialist team but increase it for front-line staff. It may be possible to identify a 'trade-off'. For example, nursing staff expressed concerns at reintroduction of placement of fine-bore feeding tubes with guidewires within their role, exclusively a medical responsibility for some years. Where would they find time to do anything more? However, they also complained about the effort required to persuade medical teams to re-site displaced feeding tubes, viewed by them as low priority, especially when 'on call'. Checking placement via mandatory chest X-ray was labour-intensive; for doctors signing requests and returning to view the X-ray films, porters and nurses in transporting the patient to and from the X-ray department and for radiographers. Gaining responsibility for siting tubes could therefore be portrayed as labour-saving, especially when linked with new placement checking procedures based on nurses checking the pH of gastric aspirate. The exploration of these concerns opened avenues to address them.

Users' views

Service users' views are equally important; clients often 'knew jolly well what they wanted from and liked about the service but were not usually asked' (Bignell, personal communication). Exploring patients' and carers' views of stroke rehabilitation, Kelson & Ford (1998) identified their overwhelming need for information – about the stroke itself, its effects, about management plans and what will happen or is available after discharge. Asking patients about their meal experiences highlighted problems (e.g. with ethnic diets and limited choice for some dietary requirements at the evening meal) but also strengths. Missing meals due to investigations/procedures, commonly cited as a problem in the literature, did not occur (Perry et al 2000).

Direct involvement in each stage of the process of change may be difficult, for example, in contributing to the development of evidence-based guidelines it may be unrealistic to ask patients or carers to participate in reviewing and critiquing the literature. They could however be asked to generate a list of questions that should be asked of the literature, be included in discussions about proposed changes, and be asked to evaluate the changes. Methods for involving service users in guideline development are discussed in Chapter 8.

'The way we do things round here'

This entails putting together a picture of organisational culture at team, ward or unit level as well as Trust-wide. Most nurses will be familiar with the marked differences in character encountered even between adjacent wards sharing consultants and patient intake. As an 'incomer' Perry et al (2000, page 17) used the Assessment of Ward Environment Schedule (Nolan et al 1998) to gauge the climate of different wards; noticeable differences appeared in staff perceptions of their recognition and regard, working relationships, team climate and workload. One ward was revealed with high scores for team-working, recognition and regard, and working relationships coinciding with lower dissatisfaction with workload. This was an admissions ward with very high levels of patient and staff activity. It also boasted earliest and highest compliance with the new guidelines, highlighting the significance of local climate for practice development.

Implementation strategies need to be planned to match local culture and expectations. How is change usually introduced? Are staff accustomed to being told what to do or are they used to self-determination? Where does the usual managerial approach lie between the extremes of enforced compliance and self-motivated adherence? Redfern et al (2000, page 157) describe one project with a mismatch between a project leader with a personal preference to encourage and motivate working with staff who waited to be enforced because that was what they expected and was the norm in their environment. In this instance, guideline implementation was slow until the project leader matched her approach to local expectations instead of trying to change the staff to meet her ideals.

Information on previous experiences of change in the Trust will be helpful. How have previous changes been handled? How was this viewed by staff – what worked well and what problems are reported? The answers to these questions explained the cynicism encountered in one area in response to attempts to involve staff in project development. A previous communication failure over ward relocation had left staff perceiving a fait accompli where managers believed they had consulted and discussed. Efforts to include staff were redoubled rather than rejection being taken at face value.

Further information should include whether anything similar has been tried in the Trust before, and with what result. Perry et al (2000, page 38) found that a nutrition risk screening tool had been introduced a year before, with little success. However, the two wards which used it wanted to keep it, so it was decided to capitalise on and top-up previous training and relaunch the same tool. Whilst improvements in nutrition risk screening were achieved, compliance remained poor. It was postulated that rather than building on existing knowledge, relaunch may have been tainted by previous failure. Similar findings occurred across the projects, leading Redfern et al (2000, page 92) to suggest that it may be easier to generate enthusiasm for something new than to enhance or resurrect existing procedures.

By completion of this phase possible levers, supports and supporters, potential hindrances or barriers to change will have been identified. At this stage it may be worth pulling it together to highlight key points. One method is to construct a force field analysis (Lewin 1951) which entails identifying those factors that are expected to promote and support the endeavour and those that will hinder and resist it. This approach was employed prior to implementing further practice development within an existing leg ulcer service (Box 10.1; Doherty et al 2000).

Another approach, used before implementing standardised multidisciplinary assessment for older adults prior to hospital discharge (O'Tuathail et al 2000) is the SWOT analysis, where potential or actual Strengths, Weaknesses, Opportunities and Threats offered by the project to the local area are identified (Box 10.2). Both these approaches concentrate on the 'big issues' and can serve to focus activities, and as a memory aid as the project progresses. However it is also important not to lose sight of detail such as individual features of wards or teams. It may also be useful to itemise supports, drivers and obstacles for individual components of the change. For example, implementing a valid and reliable swallow screening tool was one of the components of a project addressing screening, assessment and management of nutritional risk and the wide range of eating difficulties experienced by patients with acute stroke (Table 10.1). Concise notation of key features retains detail and helps to keep track of individual threads.

Altogether, this represents a key phase for any project and time spent at this point may prevent time wasted later and avoid opposition or distress.

Box 10.1 Force field analysis (Doherty et al 2000, with permission)

Forces for change	Forces against change
Open to communication and collaboration	Previous bad experience of change in this area
Will accept and cope with small-scale change	Excessive recent change/low tolerance for change
Will co-operate if benefit can be seen in the long run	Increasing workload and high stress levels
Ground staff eager to gain skills, increase professional development	Staff shortage and skills shortage (resource constraint)
Enthusiastic teams, young, eager staff, negotiation possible	Management style, viewed as low priority care
Senior managerial and Trust Board support	Staff not motivated to provide this care; 'not interested' attitude
Desire to have more control over own practice	No feedback/incentives; no perceived need for change
May perceive relative advantage to change/	New staff not yet fully integrated into Trust; may view change as

Summary

An early priority is to identify the specific requirements for the project manager post and appoint the individual who will be responsible for driving the project through. 'Diagnostic analysis' will be an essential first step for the post-holder, prior to planning change. Information gained may include:

- The current macro-organisational context
- Identifying organisational priorities, structures and strategic plans into which the changes might fit
- Identifying the key players and opinion-leaders
- Establishing their attitudes and experiences in relation to the subject
- Accessing patients'/users' experiences and views of the topic; involving them directly where feasible

---

Box 10.2 SWOT analysis (O'Tuathail et al 2000, with permission)

Strengths	**Weaknesses**
Process to develop care focused on the patient	Implementation takes time and effort
Opportunity to develop teamwork	May be seen as yet another change
Generate multidisciplinary documentation	Yet more paperwork
Create data for audit purposes	Large project involving so many disciplines
Develop evidence-based practice	Large clinical team

Opportunities	**Threats**
Develop better outcomes for patients	Lack of time for meetings, education sessions and ever-increasing workload
Assist Trust's contracting process and image of promoting quality care	Lack of commitment from individuals or professional groups of staff
Marketing initiative regionally and nationally	Overlap with other on-going projects
Improve communication across the primary/secondary interface	Resistance to change

- Getting a feel for organisational culture at all levels
- Clarifying usual management approaches and exploring previous change experiences.

What changes are needed?

Ensuring change is based on best evidence

Implementation of research evidence into practice has been repeatedly explored in nursing and key barriers identified. A common complaint of clinical nurses in all areas is difficulty accessing and making sense of the evidence (Dunn et al 1997, Funk et al 1995, Newman et

Table 10.1 Drivers and obstacles to changing the process for screening stroke patients for dysphagia and referring to speech and language dysphagia service for full clinical assessment of swallowing

Features of swallow screening procedure	Drivers/supports for change	Obstacles to change
Current swallow screen = gag as proxy	1. Only performed by doctors 2. Variability of results 3. Speech and Language Therapists believe dysphagic patients missed 4. Speech and Language Therapist concern re inappropriate referrals	A. 'Custom & practice' B. Lack of knowledge re valid methods
Screening only undertaken by doctors	1. Often omitted or delayed 2. Nurses have to request/remind; workload 3. Delayed screening impacts patient care 4. Nurses have little first-hand knowledge of patients' swallow function	A. 'Custom & practice' B. Nurses' lack of knowledge & skills C. Concern re lack of nursing skills D. Workload – another duty for nurses E. Medical sanction required for referral to Speech and Language Therapist
Referral for speech and language dysphagia assessment requires written medical referral	1. Written referral often omitted/delayed 2. Nurses have to request/remind; workload 3. Written referral accompanied by nurses contacting Speech and Language Therapist – nurse workload 4. Omitted written referral wastes Speech and Language Therapist time 5. Delayed referral impacts patient care; concern re time spent with nil orally	A. Potential transfer of referral decision-making and hence – B. Transfer of nutrition support decision-making C. Concern re inappropriate nutrition support decision-making D. Varied level of concern re duration patients spent fasting

al 1998, Redfern et al 2000, page 48). A number of approaches have been developed to process evidence and present it to health care practitioners in brief, user-friendly formats. Care pathways are one option, allowing incorporation of research evidence into a structured framework (Wigfield & Boon 1996). On a day-by-day basis the anticipated management and progress of typical patients with specific diagnoses are mapped. Another recent initiative is that of benchmarking, whereby 'best practice' features are identified for local comparison (Pantall 2001). This approach has been incorporated into a national nursing care quality initiative (Department of Health 2001a). Both of these approaches may make use of evidence-based guidelines comprising recommendations for the interventions and care management which have been shown to produce the best outcomes for a specific situation and patient group. Recommendations are identified according to the type and strength of evidence from which they derive, hence retaining a direct link with and enabling practitioners to read the underpinning evidence if they wish.

Evidence-based guidelines encapsulate 'best practice' for the target patient group and criteria against which clinical practice and patient outcomes can be compared. This enables identification of areas of strength and practice development opportunities. For example, post-stroke nutrition management guidelines recommended that all patients admitted to hospital with acute stroke should have their swallowing ability screened; where dysphagia was suspected full clinical assessment should take place within 72 hours of admission. When practice was audited and compared with these recommendations it was found that 53% of patients had been screened with 38% of assessments occurring within the specified time period (Perry & McLaren 2000). Dysphagia screening and referral processes were highlighted as practice development topics.

Evidence-based guidelines are therefore a user-friendly means to communicate research evidence and guidance on 'best practice', encompass audit criteria and may indicate practice development topics. The first stage of guideline development (i.e. seeking robust evidence to support a practice development), starts concurrently with the 'diagnostic analysis' previously described.

Finding the evidence

For both the clinical effectiveness lead initiating a project and the individual nurse seeking help with a practice issue literature searching is a starting point. Chapter 3 addresses this in detail and this section simply reiterates the importance of making full use of all available resources. Chief of these is the local health librarian who may help with accessing relevant databases and setting up and running search strategies. Discussion with a librarian can often overcome the twin stumbling blocks of searches that find nothing or 30 000 papers. For many topics recent systematic reviews or evidence-based guidelines from well-known sources of expertise are available. However, these still may not answer every aspect of the question; for example, users' views and patients' perspectives may not have been addressed; patients studied may not be representative of the local population or the nurse's case-load. Further searching for relevant evidence will be required.

Appraising the evidence

Practice recommendations or guidelines are only as good as the evidence on which they rest, and the manner in which this has been handled. Irrespective of the source of the evidence, it is important to appraise and critique the literature. Key questions to ask include:

- whether the design and methodology adopted by a study is an appropriate means to answer the particular question
- whether the methods used by the study match quality criteria required for that particular design
- whether limitations of study design and methods have been acknowledged and taken into account when results are used to produce recommendations.

Chapters 4–7 deal with this process in detail, and provide information about appropriate appraisal instruments.

Even if what appears to be evidence-based guidelines have been identified, it is important to evaluate their merits, not least because some topics have been repeatedly addressed. An American source of critically appraised guidelines, the National Guideline Clearing house (found at www.guideline.gov/), accessed in March 2001, yielded five guidelines focusing on pressure damage or ulceration, seven on continence and 14 for acute pain management. Chapter 8 discusses an appraisal instrument that can be used as a checklist or *aide-mémoire* for guideline developers or groups undertaking local modification of national guidelines. This option, tailoring nationally developed guidelines to suit local circumstances, has been commended by the NHS Executive (1996) and may offer the twin benefits of minimising time spent on literature searching and appraisal whilst maximising input of local clinicians to ensure guidelines address local circumstances and needs.

Turning evidence into recommendations

The process of developing and grading recommendations according to the strength of evidence has been discussed in Chapter 8. Recommendations that are based on evidence with a very low risk of bias are assigned a high grade. There is, however, limited availability of good-quality data in many important areas of care. In addition, the applicability of findings from controlled studies to patients in a specific clinical setting may be questionable, especially where studies have concentrated on specific subgroups. Doherty et al (2000, page 15) discuss working with a heterogeneous patient case-load with multiple risk factors resulting in only 35% of their ulcers being of purely venous origin. However, the evidence base underpinning leg ulcer management is predominantly focused on venous leg ulcers. In this and many other situations guidelines and advice may be needed most where evidence is weak or lacking.

Many topic areas are only addressed via anecdote, description, prescription and discussion. These nonetheless frequently represent important areas of patient care which are the subject of everyday treatment and management decisions. In these situations guidance is still required, perhaps to a greater degree than where strong evidence is in the public domain. The option here is to use opinion derived from clinical experience and experts in the field. This may be available in the form of consensus statements from working parties, standing committees and conference meetings, e.g. for stroke management, prior to the development of evidence-based guidelines, 'best evidence' was derived from a published consensus statement agreed at an international conference (Aboderin & Venables 1996). Where even this does not exist, consensus agreement can be sought using formal methods such as the nominal group process or Delphi technique (see Chapter 8) or consensus development panels (Bowling 1997, pages 362–365). Modified nominal group process was used to develop guidelines for pressure damage (Rycroft-Malone 2000). This entailed participants rating statements derived from the literature on the basis of their expertise and the quality and strength of the evidence. The distribution of responses was presented, discussed and statements re-rated; recommendations were drafted reflecting and indicating extent of agreement. For the guidelines for nutrition support, a consensus development panel was brought together; representation from all relevant areas of local expertise agreed local guidance for timing of initiation of artificial nutrition support in patients with unsafe swallow post stroke (Perry et al 2000). Whilst a major multicentre trial was in progress, there was no clear evidence for optimal timing.

Using the full range of evidence (but selecting a lower level of evidence only when there is no valid primary research using an appropriate study design) in the development and presentation of guidelines, allows aggregation of data from a variety of sources (from systematic review to expert opinion) in a concise format which acknowledges and identifies its origins. Not only is this transparency a quality criteria in guideline development, it is also important for implementation.

Establishing key objectives

Comparing baseline to guideline-supported practice

As indicated by Cluzeau et al (1999) rigorous guidelines identify clear standards or targets and define measurable outcomes that can be monitored. With this in mind, before proceeding to plan changes in practice it is useful to carry out a baseline evaluation of current practice for later comparison. Clinical audit staff are a useful resource here, and may guide the choice of data and manner of collection. Much information is routinely collected within organisations. Whilst there may be some difficulties about the manner in which it is presented (e.g. data on length of hospital stay may only be recorded as finished consultant episodes) and detail and accuracy (e.g. diagnostic coding; Stegmayr & Asplund 1992) what is required may be available without additional data collection. However, this information may not be routinely collected or it may be that additional effort and resources are warranted to achieve greater accuracy/relevance. Audit and data collection techniques are beyond the scope here but texts are available in most health libraries.

A baseline audit will also enable identification and prioritisation of areas of guideline-related practice where changes are required. With depiction of baseline practice and outcomes established there is a means to evaluate the effects of guideline implementation via later repetition of the data collection exercise. This is essential if the organisation is to learn what has been gained from this process. Repeat evaluation may also be a useful 'selling' point for the change management strategy; on the basis that changes will be fully evaluated it may be possible to win provisional support where it would not otherwise be forthcoming.

With standards and outcomes clarified, the next stage entails identifying guideline components that require active intervention to enable staff to meet the specified standards and outcomes. For example, the objectives that were identified and addressed to enable nurses to screen stroke patients' swallowing ability on admission to hospital are set out in Box 10.3. The processes that will accomplish identified objectives need to be considered in the light of requirements for guideline dissemination (making sure that all relevant practitioners are aware of the guidelines and their contents) and the change management process (persuading/facilitating/supporting/ensuring practice change).

Summary

Identifying practice development objectives and achievable outcomes entails:

- Accessing and appraising the evidence in relation to the characteristics of the patient group for which it will be used
- When developing guidelines or modifying national guidelines to meet local requirements, presenting the evidence as practice recommendations appropriate to the strength of supporting information
- Where evidence is lacking, consensus expert opinion can be recruited
- Identifying and auditing current practice and outcomes
- Establishing topics or standards to be addressed via guideline implementation; outcomes that will be monitored
- Pinpointing interventions and activities required to support and enable staff to implement guideline recommendations.

Box 10.3 Objectives to be met to enable nurses to screen stroke patients' swallowing ability (Perry et al 2000, with permission)

- Identification of nurses' education and training requirements
- Development of a package to meet these, including theoretical and practical instruction and assessment
- Nomination of educators and assessors
- Agreement of competence criteria
- Location of the new role within the framework of nursing competencies within the Trust
- Location of the new training package within the framework of in-service training within the Trust
- Multiprofessional agreement to nurses' performance of a previously exclusively medical role
- Identification and agreement of changes to the referral process to access full clinical assessment by dysphagia-trained speech and language therapists for patients screened by nurses.

How to implement the changes

Developing a dissemination and implementation strategy

By this stage the guidelines will have been developed and activities required to prepare staff identified. The next stage entails considering how to inform and motivate practitioners for the practice change.

If the proposed changes are small and localised the nurse may not need an elaborate implementation strategy. However, it is always wise to think the process through from all angles before launching into change. It is important to ensure that potential implications for any other areas of practice have been considered.

For a large guideline requiring a lot of preparation for implementation (for example a guideline for nutritional support, involving nursing and medical teams, therapy departments and catering and continuing beyond hospital discharge) it might be beneficial to stage the launch and address components incrementally. If it is to be introduced across a large area, a rolling programme (perhaps one ward or team at a time) may allow focused intensive input. In both these situations early limited successes may be achieved and seen to be achieved, thus encouraging practitioners and supporting the implementation process. However, there are time implications; incremental implementation may take longer although perhaps achieve better compliance. As projects running within milestones dictated by an external evaluation framework the STEP projects were not able to explore these options.

General approaches to managing change

A range of approaches can be taken when planning change (see also Chapter 9). Grol (1997) talks of *educational approaches* which derive from striving for professional competence, clearly demonstrated in the linkage of continuing professional development (CPD) with educational sessions, ranging in style from didactic lectures to workshop and small group discussions. Appealing to clinicians as rational beings, *epidemiological stances* focus on the presentation of the evidence, e.g. in the form of guidelines, and stress the scientific merits of a new course of action. The validity, reliability, credibility and presentation of the evidence is therefore key. Implementation can also be viewed as the *marketing of a product, information or strategies* that will be useful for clinicians; both the presentation of the product and the channels of information will be important. *Behavioural* change may also be utilised, underpinned by classical theories of conditioning of behaviour reliant on the influence of specific stimuli before or after the desired actions, for example, audit and feedback or performance review. It may also be possible to incorporate reminders, for example from patients, tagged to notes or built into software, e.g. for clinic review, hospital admission or discharge procedures. *Social interactionism* capitalises on the essential gregariousness of human culture, including workplace society; the influence of fellow practitioners and patients is recognised. Opinion leaders, role models, patient pressure, peer support and group norms are all acknowledged agents or resistors of change. Moving from individual to *organisational approaches*, quality care is seen as dependent upon a cascade of interrelated actions which can be supported or hindered by the structures of the organisation itself. This approach is reflected in attitudes towards adverse incidents in moving away from individual fault-finding towards a systems approach (Department of Health 2000b).

Each of these approaches offers different avenues and strategies for guideline implementation and change management. It is not envisaged that any one will meet all requirements; a combination tailored to individual situations and needs is recommended (NHS CRD 1999).

Specific approaches to managing change

At this stage, the project co-ordinator/manager will need to check that:

- Realistic goals and time frames have been set.
- Resources are sufficient. Redfern et al (2000, pages 157 and 161) suggest that it may be unreasonable to expect projects to be cost-neutral throughout; it may be more realistic to anticipate some degree of investment which will be recouped later. For all STEP projects, resourcing was an issue; projects where the patients' health status was eventually shown to have been improved significantly by the intervention all requested and received additional funding. The level was not great (approximately £2500 each; for example to fund bank nurse and locum speech and language therapists' time, see Box 10.4) and a cost–benefit analysis case study of the stroke nutrition project indicates that the investment repaid.
- Opportunities have been taken to pilot changes where possible.
- Interim review points have been identified with flexibility built in to enable changes if necessary in light of progress.
- The manager/co-ordinator role is enabled to fulfil required activities.
- Review dates for guideline implementation and for the guidelines themselves have been set.

Information from the 'diagnostic analysis' will be invaluable in guiding the choice of implementation strategies from those which have been demonstrated to achieve successful results (see also Chapter 9). Even where change is on a small scale, and no formal analysis undertaken, it is beneficial to draw on knowledge of the structures, characters, characteristics, promoting and limiting factors within the change area. Irrespective of the scale of change the key principle of matching specific strategies to achieve individual objectives applies. Relevant information might include:

- Existing initiatives within the Trust which can support the changes (e.g. for a breastfeeding initiative, where the Trust was seeking UNICEF UK Baby Friendly Hospital status)
- Existing structures within the Trust which can accommodate the changes (e.g. nursing and medical in-service training programmes)
- Interprofessional interpretation and prioritisation of key activities (e.g. nursing and medical attitudes towards siting of fine-bore feeding tubes)
- The attitudes and beliefs of key figures and groups, to guide the targeting and presentation of information
- The ward, team or Trust climate, guiding choice of appropriate approach to change from encouragement to enforcement, persuasion to compulsion
- Supportive forces that can be relied upon; resistance factors that need to be addressed
- Anticipated costs; availability of funding.

Interventions should be accommodated within existing structures where possible and strategies tailored to fit individual needs and the culture of the organisation. Box 10.4 gives a worked example.

Box 10.4 Example

The problem
In one acute Trust, swallow screening on admission of patients with stroke was a medical role with written medical referral required for full clinical assessment of swallowing by members of a speech and language dysphagia service. In practice, only around half of all patients admitted with acute stroke had their swallowing screened; screening was predominantly via non-valid methods; the referral process could be protracted (Perry & McLaren 2000). Good facilities were undermined by suboptimal processes, reflected in patient and carer complaints and staff dissatisfaction (Table 10.1).

The proposed solution
Screening by nurses. This change had been originally identified via a broad consultation process involving all grades of relevant practitioners, patients and carers.

Box 10.4 (*contd.*)

Planning the change

This entailed several steps (Table 10.2)

1. Identification of a valid and reliable method of screening swallowing function. This was undertaken by a consensus development panel chosen as the opinion leaders of their professions. Elements of the epidemiological approach were evident in choice of tool and manner of presentation, exemplifying a rigorous process expressed in clear and user-friendly documentation. Incorporation of the tool within the stroke pathway and proforma was intended to act as a visual prompt for medical and nursing staff during admission procedures. Costs of this component entailed time of project team members, photocopying and library costs accessing literature. The project manager's salary was an additional cost, funded through regional research funding streams. All other costs were subsumed within normal Trust budgets.

2. Education and training of nursing and medical staff to use this screening tool. In addition to practical preparation interventions aimed to ensure professional acceptance of new role activities, e.g. nurses siting and checking placement of feeding tubes; doctors using new screening procedures. For nurses, training sessions were accommodated within the established Scope of Professional Practice programme, comprising educational input and skills training in aspects considered core role functions of the nursing grades. Ward leaders and influential senior staff were encouraged to attend first sessions. Preparation combined theory and practice away from the ward with a minimum of five practical sessions conducted on their wards screening real patients. In addition to teaching and assessing nurses' skills, this aimed to insert the behaviour into its natural context, to associate it with daily nursing practice. Junior doctors' teaching occurred within their regular weekly programme. Costs of this component derived from extra study time required for nurses and time spent on teaching delivered by speech and language therapists and in-service trainers. Project time pressures enforced rapid implementation; this entailed use of some additional bank nurses to provide cover and locum speech and language therapy time.

Box 10.4 (*contd.*)

3. Changes in role remit enabling nurses to contact the dysphagia service with details of patients with swallowing problems. Superficially an organisational change, recruiting support for this entailed multiple approaches. Audit and feedback of baseline practice highlighted aspects for change. Local consultants, nationally acknowledged for work in this area, addressed local clinicians and chaired discussion sessions. The intervention was widely promoted; at ward and team meetings, in internal and neighbouring Trust newsletters, the local newspaper, cable TV; and at local, national and international conferences. The Trust Board and internal professional groups circulated statements of support; influential figures role-modelled changed practice. Members of the stroke team and the project manager monitored and reported progress. The costs of this component were represented largely by project manager time, photocopying and two fees for external lecturers.

Summary

- A range of approaches to change management and a variety of strategies have been shown to be effective for guideline implementation.
- Approaches and strategies need to be planned to achieve their objectives within the context of the individual organisation.
- No one approach will be adequate alone; mix and match to meet individual requirements.
- Ensure that resourcing and management issues have been addressed; goals and time frames are realistic and review dates set.

Evaluating the progress and effects of the changes

It is important to maintain close contact with the progress of implementation interventions. Be prepared to make changes if things do not work as expected. For example, the practical swallow screening sessions were originally planned to take place whenever

Table 10.2 Strategies employed to implement swallow screening guidelines

Requirements *prior to implementation*	Strategies *employed to address this*
Identification of a valid and reliable swallow screening tool	1. Consensus development panel composed of all relevant groups 2. Consensus development panel comprised opinion leaders of the professions 3. Choice of tool with demonstrated validity and reliability, including with nurses 4. Presentation of the tool within guidelines developed by rigorous process 5. Clarity and user-friendliness of format 6. Incorporation within care pathway and proforma as visual prompts
Education and training required to use the tool	1. Sessions incorporated within established uni-professional education programmes This facilitated access to staff and supported identification of screening as role 'norm' 2. Sessions function as discussion for a re role changes 3. Nurses' practical sessions take place on their wards; facilitates access to staff and associates screening with routine nursing practice 4. Ward sisters/charge nurses and senior staff encouraged to achieve competence and role model changed practice
Changes in role remit to enable nurses to alert the dysphagia service of patients needing full clinical swallowing assessment	1. Support indicated via widespread consultation process, grassroots to management levels 2. Audit and feedback of baseline working of the referral system; identification of problems 3. Recruitment of support for changing referral system from all consultants; 1:1 discussions 4. Input and discussion session with nationally acknowledged opinion leader 5. Overt and widespread high level support for changes expressed via public statements, memos and role modelling 6. 'Selling' the project through internal and local media, nationally and internationally 7. Implementation within evaluation framework allows assessment of merit of changes

therapists were on the ward seeing patients. This proved unworkable; it was not possible to co-ordinate the activities of therapists' with those of nursing staff and tie them in with patient needs on an opportunistic basis. This was changed to a programme of timed appointments; although it entailed administration time, this was successful.

Maintain the focus on sustainability. Project activities should shift from being seen as something different and special to everyday practice. Ways to address this will have been identified from the outset and include use of existing structures and processes, and involvement of clinical staff in all aspects. Members of the health care team can be encouraged to assume responsibility for project activities within their areas of practice, and, as time progresses, the role of the project manager will need to change to reflect this. Whilst it is important that someone takes responsibility to drive dissemination and implementation of the guidelines, continued reliance upon a single individual weakens the long-term sustainability of guideline-supported practice. Withdrawal of the manager should be planned, possibly around a staged progress of relinquishing responsibilities with further evaluation of guideline activities and outcomes once this has occurred.

Once formal evaluation of the changes has occurred ensure that the information is disseminated to everyone involved. Public recognition should be given for the time, energy and commitment of those who made things happen. Consider wider publication of both the processes experienced and results achieved; what has been learnt about the process of change may be as valuable to colleagues as the effects for patient care. Avenues to disseminate findings include local and national conferences, fora and interest group meetings, papers and publications ranging from major international journals to society newsletters. There are also implementation fora, e.g. Impact, a section of Bandolier, accessible on-line at www.ebandolier.com and via the NeLH.

In conclusion

This chapter has sought to draw together information covered in preceding pages and illustrate how this has been applied within real-life projects. Examples drawn from the STEP projects have been used extensively to demonstrate things which worked and pitfalls to avoid. It would be misleading to suggest that following the processes detailed guarantees success; changing practice is never easy and no two situations are identical. However, in the world of practice development there is a wealth of experience to draw on, and some of the outcomes of the STEP projects (Box 10.5) demonstrate that efforts to implement practice that is explicitly evidence-based may be well rewarded.

Box 10.5 Changes effected by the STEP projects

- Significant gains in staff knowledge and positive attitude change towards family intervention for schizophrenia
- Significant reduction in work-related psychological distress
- Increased information delivered antenatally re infant feeding
- Increased skin-to-skin contact
- Increased continuance of breast feeding to 12 weeks
- In stroke rehabilitation, significant improvements in multidisciplinary involvement and communication with carers
- Dramatic reductions in average costs of leg ulcer dressings per patient per week
- Improvements in numbers of patients with ulcers healed in 1–3 months and 3–6 months
- More complete assessment of continence problems in elderly patients
- Significant increases in nurses' knowledge of incontinence and its management
- Increased reportage of information given, involvement and satisfaction of older people with the discharge process
- Significant improvements in appropriate referrals for nutritional support; faster referral processes
- Significant reduction in time spent with nil orally prior to institution of nutrition support and throughout patient stay
- Fewer feeding tubes and X-rays required, feed quantities delivered closer to prescription
- Significant reduction in incidence of infective episodes – chest and urinary tract, sepsis of unidentified origin.

References

Aboderin I, Venables G 1996 Stroke management in Europe. Pan European Consensus Meeting on Stroke Management. Journal of Internal Medicine 240(4): 173–180

ACHCEW (Association for Community Health Councils for England and Wales) 1997 Hungry in hospital? London: ACHCEW

Bignell V, Getliffe K, Forester L 2000 The South Thames Evidence-based Practice Project. The promotion of continence for elderly people in primary care: the role of community nurses. London: St George's Hospital Medical School & Kingston University

BMA (British Medical Association) 1999 Withholding and withdrawing life-prolonging medical treatment. Guidance for decision making. London: BMJ Publishing

Bowling A 1997 Research methods in health. Buckingham: Open University Press

Clinical Standards Advisory Group 1998 Report on clinical effectiveness using stroke as an example. London: The Stationery Office

Cluzeau F, Littlejohns P, Grimshaw J, Feder G, Moran S 1999 Development and application of a generic methodology to assess the quality of clinical guidelines. International Journal of Quality in Health Care 11(1): 21–28. See also http://www.sghms.ac.uk/depts/phs/hceu/clinguid.htm

Department of Health 2000a Research and development for a first class service. R & D funding in the new NHS. Leeds: Department of Health

Department of Health 2000b An organisation with a memory: report of an expert group on learning from adverse events in the NHS. At http://www.doh.gov.uk /orgmemreport/index.htm. Accessed 26 March 2001

Department of Health 2001a The essence of care. Patient-focused benchmarking for health care practitioners. At http://www.doh.gov.uk/essenceofcare.htm. Accessed 12 March 2001

Department of Health 2001b The national service framework for older people. At http://www.doh.gov.uk/nsf/olderpeople.htm. Accessed 27 March 2001

Doherty D, Ross F, Yeo L et al 2000 The South Thames Evidence-based Practice Project. Leg ulcer management in an integrated service. London: St George's Hospital Medical School & Kingston University

Dunn V, Crichton N, Roe B, Seers K, Williams K 1997 Using research for practice: a UK experience of the BARRIERS scale. Journal of Advanced Nursing 26(6): 1203–1210

Funk SG, Tornquist EM, Champagne MT 1995 Barriers and facilitators of research utilisation. Nursing Clinics of North America 30(3): 395–407

Grol R 1997 Beliefs and evidence in changing clinical practice. British Medical Journal 315: 418–421

Intercollegiate Working Party for Stroke for the Royal College of Physicians of London 2000 National clinical guidelines for stroke. http://www.rcplondon/ pubs/ceeu_stroke. Accessed 07 June 2000

Kelson M, Ford C and the Intercollegiate Working Party for Stroke 1998 Stroke rehabilitation. Patient and carer views. London: Royal College of Physicians and College of Health

Lewin K 1951 Field theory in social science. New York: Harper

Love C, McLaren S, Smits M 2000 The South Thames Evidence-based Practice Project. Nutritional management for patients with acute stroke. London: St George's Hospital Medical School & Kingston University

Miller C, Scholes J, Freeman P 1999 Evaluation of the 'assisting clinical effectiveness' programme. In: Humphris D, Littlejohns P (eds) Implementing clinical guidelines. A practical guide. Oxford: Radcliffe Press

Newman M, Papadopoulos I, Sigsworth J 1998 Barriers to evidence-based practice. Clinical Effectiveness in Nursing 2: 11–20

NHS CRD (NHS Centre for Reviews and Dissemination) 1999 Getting evidence in to practice. Effective Health Care 5: 1

NHS Executive 1996 Clinical guidelines. Using clinical guidelines to improve patient care within the NHS. Leeds: NHSE

Nolan M, Grant G, Brown J, Nolan J 1998 Assessing nurses' work environment: old dilemmas, new solutions. Clinical Effectiveness in Nursing 2: 145–156

O'Tuathail C, Ross F, Stubberfield D 2000 The South Thames Evidence-based Practice Project. Standardised multidisciplinary assessment of older people on discharge from hospital. London: St George's Hospital Medical School & Kingston University

Pantall J 2001 Benchmarking in health care. NT Research 6(2): 568–580

Perry L, McLaren S 2000 An evaluation of implementation of evidence-based guidelines for dysphagia screening and assessment following acute stroke: phase 2 of an evidence-based practice project. Journal of Clinical Excellence 2: 147–156

Perry L, McLaren S, Bennett M 2000 The South Thames Evidence-based Practice Project. Nutritional support for patients with acute stroke. London: St George's Hospital Medical School & Kingston University

Redfern S, Christian S, Murrells T et al 2000 Evaluation of change in practice: South Thames Evidence-based Practice Project (STEP). London: King's College

Ross F, McLaren S 2000 The South Thames Evidence-based Practice Project. An overview of aims, methods and cross-case analysis of nine implementation projects. London: St George's Hospital Medical School & Kingston University

Royal College of Physicians/British Geriatrics Society 1992 Standardised assessment scales for older people. London: Royal College of Physicians/British Geriatrics Society

Rycroft-Malone J 2000 Pressure ulcer risk assessment and prevention. London: Royal College of Nursing. At http://www.rcn.org.uk/services/promote/clinical/ulcer_risk.pdf Accessed 27 March 2001

Sackett DL, Richardson WS, Rosenberg W, Haynes RB 1997 Evidence-based medicine. How to practice and teach EBM. New York: Churchill Livingstone

Stegmayr B, Asplund K 1992 Measuring stroke in the population. Quality of routine statistics in comparison with a population-based stroke registry. Neuroepidemiology 11: 204–213

Upton T, Brooks B 1995 Managing change in the NHS. London: Kogan Page

Wigfield A, Boon E 1996 Critical care pathway development: the way forward. British Journal of Nursing 5 (12): 732–735

Further reading

Easton N, Getliffe K, Mundy K 2000 The South Thames Evidence-based Practice Project. Rehabilitation care options for stroke patients. London: St George's Hospital Medical School & Kingston University

Grant J, Fletcher M, Warwick C 2000 The South Thames Evidence-based Practice Project. Supporting breastfeeding women. London: St George's Hospital Medical School & Kingston University

Lancashire S, Gournay K, Firn S et al 2000 The South Thames Evidence-based Practice Project. Disseminating family intervention for schizophrenia in routine clinical practice. London: St George's Hospital Medical School & Kingston University

Perry L 2001 Screening swallowing function of patients with acute stroke: part one: identification, implementation and initial evaluation of a screening tool for use by nurses. Journal of Clinical Nursing 10(4): 463–473

Perry L 2001 Screening swallowing function of patients with acute stroke: part two: detailed evaluation of the tool used by nurses. Journal of Clinical Nursing 10(4): 474–481

Perry L, Love CP 2001 Screening for dysphagia and aspiration in acute stroke: a systematic review. Dysphagia 16(1): 1–12

Tarpey A, Gould D, Rhodes V 2000 The South Thames Evidence-based Practice Project. Management of pressure areas in the acute setting. London: St George's Hospital Medical School & Kingston University

11

How clinical evidence can change nursing policies

Rhona Hotchkiss and Mandie Sunderland

Key points

- Developments in health care policy
- The advent of clinical governance
- Policy directives to ensure
  - comparable standards of health care
  - comparable access to health care
- Policies for nursing practice

Introduction

The existence of a theory–practice gap in nursing has been the subject of much research and discussion over the past few years (Hunt 1996). That what is known should differ from what is done, and vice versa, is sadly a doggedly persistent feature of nursing practice. The reasons why individual nurses fail to change their practice in the light of research evidence are well documented (Hunt 1996) and include poor dissemination of information about new or best practice; lack of access-related resources such as libraries, time, critical appraisal skills; and local resistance to change.

But what of the possibility of another gap: the evidence–policy gap? Does evidence about clinical practice shape health care policies? Do policies influence the way that health professionals practice? In exploring this topic, we have drawn solely from examples of strategies for evidence-based policy that are evolving within the United Kingdom, however similar moves to introduce evidence-based policies exist in other countries.

A strict definition of health and/or nursing policy might incorporate only those documents formulated within health departments and on occasion made public in the form of government Green

Papers which, when approved by parliament, become White Papers and enter statute. This kind of policy, though, rarely deals directly with clinical care, but instead gives direction to the health service at a broader organisational level, usually focusing on the extent and methods of investment by the government.

The *Concise Oxford Dictionary* defines policy in fairly broad terms as 'A course or principle of action adopted or proposed by a government, party, business, or individual etc.' If we widen our definition of policy to include direction given by any body sanctioned by government through the health departments, we reach the level at which decisions are taken that have a direct influence on how, where, why and by whom clinical care is delivered; the level at which most practitioners will experience the direct influence of policy. It is under this broader umbrella definition of 'policy' that the influence of clinical evidence will be considered here.

Individual patient care and the decisions required about interventions to facilitate patient movement along an optimum pathway have been the subject of much activity in health care over the last two decades in particular. The utilisation of clinical evidence at this level is a separate sphere from the use of clinical evidence to affect policy decisions. Policy decisions are usually made by people in settings remote from the level of individual patient care and involve dealing with, and legislating for, generalisable situations.

Although there will, inevitably, be time gaps between the issuing of new policy that aims to promulgate the latest clinical evidence and consequent changes in practice, and between the generation of clinical evidence and its having an effect on policy development, the absolute necessity of that relationship between policy and clinical evidence cannot be overstated.

The health service needs policy and, most vitally, patient care needs policy that:

- Is informed by evidence
- Gives unequivocal support to the principle of comparable standards of evidence-based care across health care organisations
- Makes the routine application of evidence-based care easier, incorporating an active attempt to dismantle barriers to the generation and use of evidence about clinical practice.

If existing health service policy is fashioned with these aims in mind, it should be possible to see clear themes relating to the use of clinical evidence running through policy documents. What is required is that a circular relationship of evidence-affecting-policy-affecting-practice is visible in the language of, and actions arising from, policy documents. So how does current health policy shape up against this standard?

Evidence-based policy at a regional level: the UK model

Policy for health care which will exert an influence on clinical practice over the coming 5–10 years varies between the UK regions of England, Scotland, Wales and Northern Ireland and, since devolution, has arguably become more divergent in response to differing 'local' priorities.

Prior to 1999, all legislative power for the four regions was held by the Westminster Parliament in London. Despite this, each of the four regions had its own health department/executive and its own chief nursing and medical officers. In 1999, Scotland elected its own parliament with almost full legislative power for matters pertaining to Scotland, including health (but excluding a few areas such as defence, which remained a matter for the UK parliament). Wales and Northern Ireland elected members to their own National Assemblies with somewhat less legislative power than the Scottish Parliament, but nevertheless with the ability to make decisions about health care in Wales and Northern Ireland.

Although there have always been regional differences in health care decision-making and provision in the UK health system, the rapidly evolving situation presented by devolution presents an interesting conundrum for the UK National Health Service. In theory, standards in service provision and quality could vary widely between the regions in response to local drivers for change. For example public opinion about priorities for spending or differing political sensitivities may dictate spending locally. However, where clinical evidence dictates health policy, there should be a degree of uniformity. The potential for services to improve across the UK through the increasing opportunity for benchmarking (i.e. the comparing of performance and sharing of best practice and innovative solutions) that devolution provides, should ensure that policy is driven by clinical evidence. For example it would be difficult to justify a situation where a particular medication was being made available in Wales or England because of the associated evidence base, but not in Northern Ireland or Scotland.

Devolution and its impact on the organisation and delivery of health services is in its infancy and measurements of net gains in the quality of clinical care will not be possible for some years to come.

Since being elected in 1997, and re-elected in June 2001 in the UK, the Labour administration has made clear its over-riding priority to modernise the NHS. As a result, a wide range of policy documents has been produced aimed at enabling the reorganisation of health services to tackle major health inequalities. The focus of this chapter will be on selected policy examples from England and Scotland where, because of sheer numbers and the impact of devolved parliament status respectively, policy-making activity has been greatest. Key examples of policy and policy-related initiatives in health care include:

■ England: *A First Class Service: Quality in the New NHS* including Clinical Governance and National Service Frameworks (Department of Health 1998), the National Institute for Clinical Excellence (NICE) and The Commission for Health Improvement (CHI)

■ Scotland: *Designed to Care* including the Nursing and Midwifery Practice Development Unit (Scottish Office Department of Health 1997), *The Acute Services Review* including Managed Clinical Networks and the Clinical Standards Board for Scotland (Scottish Office Department of Health 1998).

Clinical governance

Designed to Care (Scottish Office Department of Health 1997) in Scotland and *A First Class Service* (Department of Health 1998) in England introduced the concept of clinical governance to the NHS. While the term 'clinical governance' *per se* may have been new to the NHS, the pursuit of clinical quality was not. Clinical governance is defined in *A First Class Service* as:

A framework through which NHS organisations are accountable for continuously improving the quality of their services and safeguarding high standards of care by creating an environment in which excellence and clinical care will flourish. (page 4)

The central tenet of clinical governance is that quality of clinical care – and by implication care that is evidence-based – is to be the driving factor behind decisions about service delivery. This new 'duty of quality' requires all NHS organisations to put in place arrangements for monitoring and improving the quality of the health care they provide.

To those involved in service delivery within the NHS, what the introduction of clinical governance means in practice is that:

- clear lines of responsibility and accountability must be introduced to ensure the overall quality of clinical care
- a comprehensive programme of quality improvement activities must be implemented
- procedures must be put in place for all professional groups to identify and remedy poor performance.

Guidance to the NHS, Clinical Governance: Quality in the New NHS (Scottish Office Department of Health 1999) provides a framework for the implementation of clinical governance. It outlines a vision for the next 5 years leading to a single, coherent, local programme for quality improvement. It intends this to be achieved through:

- An open and participative culture in which education, research and the sharing of good practice are expected and valued
- Commitment to quality at all levels and in all groups within NHS organisations
- An ethos of working closely with patients, users, carers and the public
- Commitment on the part of the boards of NHS organisations to quality, demonstrated by regular discussions of key issues
- Multidisciplinary working
- Good information systems and use of their products.

Designed to Care; Renewing the National Health Service in Scotland (Scottish Office Department of Health 1997) aimed to set out the direction for 'a service which is designed from the patients viewpoint, which delivers clinically-effective care and which does so quickly and reliably in high-quality facilities' (page 2). This patient-centred approach was welcomed by nurses particularly the suggestion in chapter 2, Better services for patients, that this include, 'improving clinical effectiveness by ensuring that performance meets standards and that these standards are driven upwards'.

Nurses, midwives and health visitors have a key role to play in optimising the impact of clinical governance. Nursing has a long tradition of commitment to standard-setting, care pathway development, the use of protocols and guidelines. The challenge inherent in clinical governance is to ensure that guidelines and care pathways are explicitly evidence-based and that they are applied consistently in appropriate circumstances. The Royal College of Nursing, in recognition of the extensive skill and time requirements for guideline development, has taken the initiative to prioritise and develop guidelines for a number of different aspects of care. It is up to educational institutions and health care organisations to ensure that nurses develop the relevant skills for deciding, in consultation with the patient, whether to implement recommendations from such guidelines. Research findings must be shown to be relevant to clinical practice, with nurses being offered training in critical appraisal to enable them to use research evidence to positively influence individual patient outcome. In addition, health care organisations will need to foster and facilitate an evaluative approach to patient care, instilling life-long learning habits. Many nurses have embraced the concept of evidence-based practice, however it is clear that the delivery of evidence-based care is not universal and that patients may then not always be receiving optimum care. More work is needed to ensure that nurses and midwives are provided with the necessary skills and support to make the adoption of such practice a global reality.

Policies designed to ensure comparable standards of health care across the four United Kingdom countries

The National Institute for Clinical Excellence (NICE)

The National Institute for Clinical Excellence (NICE) was established as a Special Health Authority for England in 1999. Its stated aim is to promote clinical and cost-effectiveness by providing clinical guidance and related audit methodologies to clinical staff in England and Wales. NICE will advise on the best use of existing treatments in the NHS in England and Wales, appraise new health care interventions and technologies, and advise how these can be implemented and how best they may fit alongside existing treatments. They will also incorporate the work carried out under the umbrella term of Confidential Enquiries, namely:

- Peri-operative deaths
- Still births and deaths in infancy
- Maternal deaths
- Suicide and homicide by people with mental illness.

The results of all four confidential enquiries will be fed into the production of future NICE clinical guidance.

Examples of their work to date include:

- An audit tool for use in primary care for the management of patients who have had myocardial infarction. This is the first of a range of audit support projects relevant to coronary heart disease.

- National guidelines which are either commissioned by NICE or are developed from existing guidelines, providing they fulfil preset criteria. The Secretary of State for Health and the National Assembly for Wales select the topics taking into consideration NHS priorities and National Service Frameworks (see below). Individual health care practitioners are also able to suggest guidelines to NICE via the website (http://www.nice.org.uk). Clinical effectiveness and affordability are key criteria for NICE guidelines. Guidelines are available for a range of topics such as induction of labour, head injury in children and adults, eating disorders and dyspepsia.

Prior to the establishment of NICE there was no coherent approach in England to the appraisal of research evidence and the production of guidance for clinical practice. It is intended that NICE provide a single reference point to front line clinicians on clinical standards and cost effectiveness. Information can be accessed via the above internet address or via the National Electronic Library for Health (http://www.nelh.nhs.uk).

NICE has focused mainly on medical interventions, as opposed to the broader area of health interventions; however, the publication of guidelines in relation to the prevention and management of pressure sores may signal the first of many opportunities for nurses, midwives and health visitors to ensure that the evidence they have worked to build translates into policy which in turn drives widespread change in practice.

The Acute Services Review

The Acute Services Review Report (Scottish Office Department of Health 1998) introduced several measures in an attempt to ensure the uniform application of clinical evidence across the NHS in Scotland. The report dealt with several distinct clinical topics – renal services, coronary heart disease, emergency services and others, using clinical evidence submitted by nurses to make recommendations about the redesign of these services.

Crucially, though, for the future of evidence-based health policy in Scotland, the Review set in motion the development of Managed Clinical Networks and the Clinical Standard Board for Scotland (discussed later).

Managed Clinical Networks

Managed Clinical Networks were described as being the best way for the NHS in Scotland to achieve 'equitable, rational and sustainable acute services', (Scottish Executive Department of Health 1999) which would allow for greater emphasis to be placed on performance and effectiveness.

The Networks – to incorporate representatives of the different health care professions and managers from settings including primary and secondary care, local services and tertiary referral centres – should reach agreement, based on available evidence and expertise, on protocols and pathways of treatment in relation to specific clinical conditions. The aim is to ensure that all patients receive the same standards of care regardless of their proximity to 'centres of excellence', since they should be following common treatment and care pathways across the country.

Managed Clinical Networks are in their infancy at this time, but once again offer the potential for clinical evidence to drive policy at the crucial level of designing and supporting the best possible patient journeys.

The Scottish Intercollegiate Guidelines Network (SIGN)

SIGN was established in 1993 by the Academy of Medical Royal Colleges in Scotland and exists to develop evidence-based guidelines for use in the NHS in Scotland. The network has developed over 40 guidelines to date, against an agreed and latterly revised methodology (http://www.sign.ac.uk/methodology/index.html). The SIGN programme appears to offer the potential for nurses and the nursing policy to affect and be affected by clinical evidence. However, in practice, the SIGN programme is medically dominated and their topic selection leans towards areas where there exists a substantial body of scientific evidence around treatment and interventions.

Nevertheless, SIGN does include nurses, midwives and health visitors on its development groups and in the wider consultation processes they undertake in the development process. There exists a real opportunity for clinical evidence amassing from nursing sources to impact upon these guidelines. It is important to note that the work of statutory organisations such as the Clinical Standards Board for Scotland are heavily reliant upon SIGN guidelines in the writing of the condition-specific standards that all NHS organisations must comply with.

The Nursing and Midwifery Practice Development Unit (NMPDU)

The NMPDU aims to 'concentrate on the development and promotion of clinical excellence, and encourage networking and the sharing of good practice throughout the NHS in Scotland' (Scottish Executive Department of Health 1999, page 29). The unit was launched in December 1999 with a remit to ensure that 'practice development goes ahead in Scotland on a planned and cohesive basis and that lessons learned in any area – clinical or geographical – are shared across the country to the benefit of patient care' (http://www.nmpdu.org.uk).

The NMPDU has concentrated on:

- Building a network of link nurses from every Trust and academic department in Scotland
- Establishing a database of good and innovative practice – planned, in progress or established and evaluated – accessible at http://www.nmpdu.org.uk

■ Defining priorities for the development of best practice statements for nursing and midwifery through a wide-ranging consultation process with practising nurses and midwives; priorities identified included nutrition, continence, tissue viability and communication. The approach to building best practice statements involves using evidence where it exists, building consensus based on existing good practice and highlighting areas for further research and development that units such as the Nursing Research Initiative for Scotland (NRIS) or individual practitioners may move forward on.

While the NMPDU is an NHS unit, its Director is accountable to the Chief Nursing Officer for Scotland. *Caring for Scotland: A Strategy for Nursing and Midwifery in Scotland* (Scottish Executive Health Department 2001a), gives the NMPDU responsibility for making recommendations to the Scottish Executive Health Department about new and innovative practice that has wrought a demonstrable improvement in patient care and should be considered for implementation across the country.

In these ways, the NMPDU will offer practitioners – using the clinical evidence they amass – a further opportunity to shape policy on health and specifically nursing care.

Standard setting and monitoring for quality

The Commission for Health Improvement (CHI)

The Commission for Health Improvement (CHI), established in 2000, aims to help the NHS guarantee, monitor and improve clinical care throughout England and Wales. It has a responsibility to:

■ Provide independent scrutiny of clinical governance arrangements, in the form of reviews. Hospitals undergoing review are required to provide relevant information for assessment. In addition, CHI reviewers visit the hospital to collect information about the clinical governance processes. A report outlining best practice and areas for improvement is then prepared and published on the CHI website (http://www.chi.nhs.uk)

■ Conduct and assist with investigations or enquiries into serious service failures, as appropriate

- Conduct studies to monitor and review the implementation of National Service Frameworks, NICE guidance and other key NHS policies
- Provide national leadership for the development and dissemination of clinical governance principles.

The guiding principle driving the work of the CHI is that unjustifiable variations in clinical treatment should be eradicated and that all patients get the best possible clinical care. Central to this mission is that the work of the CHI will be based on the best evidence available and will focus on improvement.

A study to identify what progress has been made nationally towards implementing improvements in cancer care highlights some of the CHI's work. Data are being collected from NHS organisations, patients and general practitioners to determine the extent to which a predetermined framework for improved cancer care has been implemented. The framework (set out in the Calman Hine report (Calman et al 1995) covers a number of principles, the implementation of which can and should be influenced by members of the nursing profession, for example:

- Providing high-quality care, in close proximity to the home where possible
- Promoting awareness of options and outcomes
- Improving communication between service providers
- Ensuring primary care involvement
- Delivering patient-centred services
- Ensuring good psychosocial care.

A sample of nurses, patients and general practitioners is being given the opportunity by the CHI to identify and communicate their experiences and views on cancer services through focus groups. In theory this should provide nurses with the opportunity to impact on cancer care policy.

In addition to national studies, such as the Cancer Care Study and a planned programme of visits involving a 4-yearly clinical governance review for every Trust in England, the CHI will be able to respond to requests from individuals and organisations that are seriously concerned about the quality of services within an organisation. Organisations can themselves invite the CHI in to advise on and help identify solutions to local difficulties.

Where the CHI is able to investigate the application of individual recommendations within NICE guidance for example, it may well become a real tool in ensuring that evidence-based practice is implemented at a local and national level across England. If the CHI is to fulfil its remit of providing independent scrutiny of clinical governance arrangements locally, procedures for implementing evidence-based nursing care will have to rank high on its list of arrangements to be scrutinised.

As with many other recent NHS policy initiatives, the value of the CHI in driving forward evidence-based care has yet to be demonstrated.

The Clinical Standards Board for Scotland

The Clinical Standards Board for Scotland (CSBS) was established in 1999 as a result of the recommendations contained within the *Acute Services Review Report* (Scottish Office Department of Health 1998). It has a unique position in UK and, some would argue, in world health care. The system of standard setting, quality assurance and accreditation for health care developed by the CSBS is the subject of worldwide interest with several European countries considering adopting its approach.

The CSBS is a statutory body, with three main functions all designed to increase public confidence in the NHS Scotland. They are:

- To set standards for clinical care
- To undertake external peer review of performance against these standards
- To report on findings.

All Trusts must comply with the CSBS standards, which are set at levels considered to be stretching but achievable.

Crucially for any examination of how clinical evidence affects policy-making, the CSBS standards will 'be based on evidence (recognising that levels and types of evidence will vary)' (Clinical Standards Board for Scotland 2001a, page 10). The standard setting groups – who also review Trust performance against standards (a model replicated by the CHI in England) – are professionally led and driven and include patient/public representatives and crucially, service users and/or their relatives who have experience of living with the condition under consideration.

Standards developed so far have included:

- Breast, colorectal, lung and ovarian cancer
- Palliative care
- Schizophrenia
- Secondary prevention following myocardial infarction.

Generic standards have also been developed, which in effect monitor the implementation of clinical governance (Clinical Standards Board for Scotland 2001a).

All of the standards relating to specific clinical conditions outline the evidence base from which they are built. Nursing and patient/ user input to the development of the evidence base for standards has been appropriately high. The evidence-base for standards for schizophrenia for example (Clinical Standards Board for Scotland 2001b) was developed with a project team of nine, including two research nurses and two psychiatrists.

The CSBS is entirely dependent upon the utilisation of clinical evidence in the development of their standards. But crucially, they consider that *evidence* should include the subjective, lived experience of patients, carers and professional health care staff. As such, they arguably represent the way forward in policy-making for clinical care in the NHS. They also provide a vehicle for nurses, midwives and health visitors to make their voice heard in an arena often seen as being dominated by RCTs that may take little account of quality of life or public acceptability issues.

National Service Frameworks (NSFs)

National Service Frameworks (NSFs) have been included in this section as their key role is that of standard setting, however they do have a broader remit:

- Setting national standards
- Establishing milestones against which performance can be measured
- Defining service models for specific services or care groups
- Addressing the 'whole system of care' which necessitates collaboration between health service providers, local authorities, the voluntary sector, and other governmental departments
- Establishing programmes to support implementation (Department of Health 1998).

In pursuit of this agenda, NSFs aim to bring together the best evidence of clinical and cost-effectiveness along with the views of patients, clients and their carers across England. The services or care groups for which NSFs are being developed include mental health, coronary heart disease, older people, diabetes, renal services, paediatric intensive care, the children's national service and cancer. The NSF for older people outlines eight key standards of care together with supporting evidence. One of the standards, promoting health and well-being, includes initiatives that range from projects such as home energy efficiency schemes and exercise services, to immunisation programmes for influenza and management of blood pressure. Implementation of these approaches will require collaboration between different agencies and professions.

The potential for clinical evidence to influence policy and for policy to support the application of evidence in practice is encouraging but as yet largely untested.

Summary

These policy initiatives are as relevant and important to nurses and midwives as they are to any other group within the NHS. They represent a multipronged approach to ensuring that clinical evidence drives clinical care, resulting in comparable practice across the UK. They also then represent the best opportunity available to nurses for influencing the direction and content of policy that determines the standards of care the NHS will be expected to work to.

In addition to these, there are also policies, strategies and initiatives that are of particular interest to nursing and midwifery and in which we should be able to appreciate the influence of evidence about nursing and from nurses.

Policy specific to nursing practice

Policy specific to nursing, midwifery and health visiting, as with more general policy initiatives, has also taken different forms in the four regions, with the following key documents being published in England and Scotland:

- England: *Making a Difference: Strengthening the nursing, midwifery and health visiting contribution to health and health care* (Department of Health 2000)

- Scotland: *Caring for Scotland: The strategy for nursing and midwifery in Scotland* (Scottish Executive Health Department 2001a) and *Nursing for Health: A review of the contribution of nurses, midwives and health visitors to improving the public's health in Scotland* (Scottish Executive Health Department 2001b).

Making a Difference

The document that will shape nursing in England over the coming 5–10 years – *Making a Difference* (Department of Health 2000) – makes specific mention of the absolute necessity for a tangible link between evidence and practice and is unequivocal in its support for the principle. Chapter 7, 'Enhancing the quality of care' (page 44) is particularly relevant and makes clear how nurses, midwives and health visitors can influence care through the assimilation of clinical evidence: 'Practice needs to be evidence-based. Research evidence will be rigorously assessed and made accessible. Nurses, midwives and health visitors need better research appraisal skills to translate research findings into practice.' Plans to grow this capacity within the professions have been outlined (Department of Health 2000).

Clinical practice benchmarking

Clinical benchmarking has been defined as 'the continuous, systematic search for and implementation of, best practices which lead to superior performance' (Pantall 2001). The intention to develop a system for clinical benchmarking for nursing in England was outlined in *Making a Difference*.

The intention was to 'explore, with the nursing, midwifery and health visiting professions, the benefits of benchmarking to examine whether it provides the best means of supporting our vision to refocus on the fundamental and essential aspects of care.' Reports by the Health Advisory Service and the Health Service Commissioner had drawn attention to poor standards in what many would regard as the 'fundamentals' of nursing care:

- Nutrition
- Hygiene and mouth care
- Tissue viability/pressure ulcers
- Continence
- Safety of clients with mental health needs

- Record keeping
- Privacy and dignity
- Principles of self-care.

In 2000, the clinical practice benchmarking initiative was launched by England's Chief Nursing Officer, Sarah Mullaly. Clinical practice benchmarking – an approach previously demonstrated to have improved patient care in NHS settings (Ellis et al 2000) – involves the development of evidence-based standards for nursing practice. For each of the key areas above, consumers and health professionals developed draft benchmarks, which were submitted to a process of consultation and review before being launched in 2001 for integration into every Trust in England. The benchmark for nutrition, for example, includes a statement reflecting an agreed patient/client outcome, and 10 key benchmarks of best practice. These benchmarks relate to factors such as providing assistance with eating and drinking, ensuring the environment is conducive for meals, availability of meals, etc.

The resulting 'pack' is a weighty and complex tome, which while well researched and presented, will require a degree of local translation if it is to be made accessible to practitioners. As always, the impact of the work will require investigation on an on-going basis as the approach evolves and is refined.

Making a Difference is on the whole, and as is common with many strategies of this kind, more about nurses than nursing; that is, it is more concerned with education, careers and professional development than with nursing care *per se*. The advent of clinical practice benchmarking though, if actively promoted and adequately supported at local level may well offer a real opportunity to close the evidence–policy–practice loop.

Caring for Scotland

Caring for Scotland (Scottish Executive Health Department 2001a) outlines the intention to ensure that the links between research, innovation and practice development are made explicit. This will be facilitated through the development of a mechanism to ensure best practice is disseminated and implemented consistently throughout Scotland.

The intention implicit within the remit of the CSBS to ensure comparable standards of care for those who use NHS services in

Scotland – wherever and whenever they access them – is also what drives the action promised in *Caring for Scotland*. Several of the action points are built on clinical evidence and are concerned with ensuring that evidence drives changes in practice:

- The development of clinical practice relating to care of children in the community
- The development of a model to develop, disseminate and implement best practice in the care of older people
- Implementation of an education package to help support workers meet the nutritional needs of older people
- Exploration of good and innovative practice in the care of people with chronic disease or enduring mental health problems
- Ensuring that where innovative practices can demonstrate improvements in patient care, they are introduced widely.

Caring for Scotland has a distinctly clinical feel to it, but as with other recent policy documents examined here, it is as yet untested and unproven. As is the case with *Making a Difference*, the Scottish strategy's best hope of closing the evidence–policy–practice loop lies in the clinically focused initiatives listed above.

Nursing for Health

Nursing for Health: A review of the contribution of nurses, midwives and health visitors to improving the public's health in Scotland (Scottish Executive Health Department 2001b) constitutes a major review of current practice and the potential future contribution of nurses to the public's health. The document incorporates examples of good and leading-edge practice, highlighting a clear link between the aspirations of the nurses involved and the emerging policy. However, the projects described neatly illustrate the inherent difficulty of providing the evidence on which to build future policy, where the outcomes of interest are in the vein of improved uptake of services, better interaction between different agencies and more contact between health professionals and vulnerable groups.

The report does, however, incorporate many recommendations which will doubtless help nurses presently working in public health settings to feel they are actively influencing policy:

- NHS Boards to facilitate the greater involvement of nurses in community planning
- School nursing to be fully integrated into Primary Care Trusts
- A new role and career pathway in public health nursing to be developed incorporating those of health visitor and school nurse
- The expertise of infection control, occupational health nurses and community psychiatric nurses to be available as resources to local health care co-operatives
- Community learning disability nurses to act as expert resources to mainstream services in meeting the needs of people with learning disability.

Once again the challenge of making these recommendations a reality remains. Producing robust clinical evidence around initiatives primarily concerned with issues of social inclusion, social justice and which involve multiagency collaboration is unlikely – at least in the short term. Nurses will have to work hard to produce evidence that will serve as a proxy for health improvement, for example increased smoking cessation, improved breastfeeding rates, a higher uptake of exercise amongst school-age children.

This kind of success will be the evidence through which nurses can shape future health policy in these complex settings.

Summary

These policies, specific to nursing, midwifery and health visiting, were developed as a collaborative exercise involving the UK Departments of Health, the professions, patient/public representatives and others working within the NHS. As such, they involve considerable compromises between the ideal and the possible. How much of this planned change – compromise though it may be – is allowed to come to fruition before being superseded by another 'better' policy remains to be seen.

Conclusion

These few select examples of 'policy' from the NHS in England and the NHS Scotland contain enough of a smattering of evidence-based action and pro-evidence language to suggest that we can be hopeful for the future of evidence-based policy. They will require to be re-visited in 5 years time with the following questions in mind:

- Do 'ordinary' practitioners feel that they have shaped and can shape policy at local and national level?
- Does policy reflect the reality of their lives and their aspirations for the future of patient care?

The ultimate test of the influence of clinical evidence on policy must surely be that if the evidence–policy–practice dialogue is truly taking place, inexplicable variations in clinical care will cease to exist.

References

Calman K et al 1995 A policy framework for commissioning cancer services. Improving the quality of cancer services. A report by the expert advisory group on cancer to the Cheif Medical Officers of England and Wales. Department of Health. http://doh.gov.uk/pub/docs/cancerfr.pdf

Clinical Standards Board for Scotland 2001a Generic standards. Edinburgh: CSBS

Clinical Standards Board for Scotland 2001b Schizophrenia. Edinburgh: CSBS Commission for Health Improvement

Department of Health 1998 A first class service: Quality in the new NHS. London: The Stationery Office

Department of Health 2000 Making a difference: strengthening the nursing, midwifery and health visiting contribution to health and healthcare. London: Stationery Office

Ellis J et al 2000 Making a difference: clinical benchmarking part 1. Nursing Standard 14(32): 33–37

Hunt J 1996 Barriers to research utilisation. Journal of Advanced Nursing 23(3): 423–425

Pantall J 2001 Benchmarking in healthcare. Nursing Times Research 6(2): 568–580

Scottish Executive Department of Health 1999 Managed clinical networks management executive letter. 10 February 1999

Scottish Executive Health Department 2001a Caring for Scotland: The strategy for nursing and midwifery in Scotland. Edinburgh: The Stationery Office

Scottish Executive Health Department 2001b Nursing for health: A review of the contribution of nurses, midwives and health visitors to improving the public's health in Scotland. Edinburgh: The Stationery Office

Scottish Office Department of Health 1997 Designed to care; Renewing the National Health Service in Scotland. Edinburgh: The Stationery Office

Scottish Office Department of Health 1998 The acute services review report. Edinburgh: The Stationery Office

Scottish Office Department of Health 1999 Guidance to the new NHS, Clinical Governance: Quality in the new NHS. Edinburgh: The Stationery Office.

Glossary

Absolute risk reduction (ARR) & increase (ARI) This figure tells us the size of the difference between outcomes in the control group and outcomes in the intervention (or exposure) group. It is the difference between the control event rate and the experimental (or exposure) event rate.

Bias Systematic error in the design, conduct or interpretation of a study. When present, it distorts the results of the study.

Blinding (masking) The method used to conceal whether or not the subject is receiving (or has received) the experimental intervention. RCTs may be classified as single-blind, double-blind, triple-blind, etc. depending on the level of blinding. For example, where both the participants and the investigators assessing the outcomes are blinded, the trial is usually classified as double-blind.

Boolean operators Used when searching electronic databases. These operators are AND, OR and NOT and are used to combine search terms.

Case control study An observational study where individuals with the target disorder (cases) and individuals without the target disorder (controls) are identified. Researchers look back in time to try and identify what factors are more prevalent in cases than controls.

CATs & CATmaker software CAT stands for critically appraised topic. These are proforma that are used to summarize the results of a critical appraisal. The Centre for Evidence Based Medicine produces CATmaker software which can be used to produce CATs and which includes the facility to use the computer to calculate figures such as the number needed to treat etc.

Clinical effectiveness This term is used in two ways. First, as shorthand for the processes used to improve the quality of health care. Secondly, to refer to the extent to which a specific clinical intervention, when deployed in the field for a particular patient or population, delivers the intended outcomes such that the benefits outweigh the harms.

Clinical governance A framework through which health care organisations are accountable for continuously improving the quality of health services and safeguarding high standards of care.

Cohort study An observational study where patients exposed to a drug or other agent are identified and followed forward in time to see whether they develop particular outcomes. People not exposed to the agent (i.e. a control group) may be included in the study.

Confidence interval (CI) Research studies use samples from the population. If the same study was carried out 100 times on different samples of the same population, 100 different results would be obtained. These results would spread around a true but unknown value. The confidence interval estimates this sampling variation. Thus we can think of the confidence interval as the range in which we can be sure that the population value lies. It is possible to calculate this range from the data obtained in a single study. By convention the 95% confidence interval is often used, i.e. the true population value will lie between these two points in 95% of cases. For example, if a study reported a difference in mortality rates between two groups as 10% with an upper 95% CI limit of 13% and lower 95% confidence limit of 7%, we know that in 95% of cases the true size of this difference is between 7% and 13%.

Confounder A factor that affects the observed relationship between the variables under investigation.

Constant comparative analysis Used in qualitative studies, the researcher constantly seeks out cases in the data set during the collection of the data that support or 'shape' provisional hypotheses.

Control event rate (CER) This is the proportion of participants in the control group in whom the outcome is observed.

Control group The control group in a study is that group of subjects who do not receive the intervention or exposure. A second group receiving the intervention or exposure can be compared against the control group.

Critical appraisal The process of systematically evaluating a piece of evidence to assess its quality, importance and applicability.

Cross-sectional study Data are collected from a representative sample of individuals at the same point in time.

Experimental event rate (EER) This is the proportion of participants in the treatment (intervention) group in whom the outcome is observed.

Incidence The number of new cases of a disease occurring in a population at risk, in a specified period of time.

Index term A controlled vocabulary term/keyword(s) used by all the indexers in an organisation to ensure consistency in assigning terms to articles on the same topic. For example, a search using the index term 'kidney transplant' also retrieves papers where the author refers to the procedure as 'renal transplant'.

Intention to treat analysis This means that study participants are analysed in the groups to which they were randomised even if they 'dropped out' or deviated from the study protocol. Intention to treat analysis mimics real life situations because it investigates the outcomes following a management decision to use a particular treatment.

Kappa coefficient (κ) A statistical test used to measure reliability. The results are reported between 0 and 1. The nearer the result is to 1, the more reliable.

Median The midpoint on a scale. Half of the observations have a value less than or equal to the median and half have a value greater than or equal to the median.

Meta-analysis Used in systematic reviews, this is the process of statistically synthesising the data from a number of studies. Meta-analysis is not appropriate in all systematic reviews.

Naturalistic enquiry Relating to qualitative research, phenomena are studied within their natural setting rather than within a superficial or controlled one. The approach aims to minimise investigator manipulation of the study setting and places no prior constraint on what the outcomes will be.

Negative case analysis Used in qualitative research, the process of actively searching for cases that appear to be inconsistent with the emerging analysis.

Negative likelihood ratio The ratio of true negative results to false negative results. A negative likelihood ratio of 0.5 means that a negative test result is half as likely to occur in patients with the condition as in patients without the condition.

Negative predictive value The proportion of people with negative test results who do not have the target disorder (should be high).

Number needed to harm The number of patients that need to be treated if an episode of harm is to occur in one person.

Number needed to treat The number of patients that need to be treated if a beneficial outcome is to occur in one person.

Odds The probability of an event happening i.e. the ratio of the number of people having the outcome of interest to the number of people not having the outcome of interest.

Odds ratio The ratio of the odds of an event in the treatment (or exposure) group compared to the odds of the event in the control (or unexposed) group.

Placebo A biologically inert substance that is sometimes given to participants in the control arm of a trial. It helps to conceal which arm of the trial the participants are in.

Positive likelihood ratio The ratio of true positive results to false positive results. A positive likelihood ratio of 8.5 means that a positive test result is 8.5 times as likely to occur in patients with the condition as in patients without the condition. (A positive likelihood ratio of 1 means that a positive test is equally as likely to occur in patients with the condition as in patients without the condition.)

Positive predictive value The proportion of people with positive test results who have the target disorder (should be high).

Prevalence This is the number of cases of the outcome of interest (e.g. a disease) in a defined population at a given point in time.

Qualitative research The meanings, experiences, practices and views of individuals are explored within their natural settings. Qualitative research aims to understand real world situations as they unfold, from the point of view of the people who live in these worlds.

Randomised controlled trial (RCT) A study in which subjects are assigned to the experimental intervention group or to the comparison group(s) by random allocation.

Reflexivity A technique used in qualitative research, especially in the analysis of data, where the author reflects on how she or he may have shaped or influenced the research findings.

Relative risk (RR) The ratio of the risk in one group compared to the other.

Relative risk reduction (RRR) The proportional reduction in rates of events between the experimental and control group.

Reliability A measure of how constant the process of data collection, coding and analysis is in a study. Test–retest reliability measures the consistency of a test on the same patient. Inter-rater reliability measures the extent to which the tests are applied consistently by different investigators in the same study.

Respondent (member) checking Used in qualitative research, the process of feeding back the researcher's interpretations of the data to informants to determine whether they recognise and agree with them.

Sample Research is carried out on a subgroup of the population. This subgroup is often referred to as the study sample. A variety of sampling methods can be employed to select the sample depending on the purpose of the research.

Sensitivity When applied to diagnostic tests, sensitivity refers to the proportion of people with a target disorder who have a positive test result.

Specificity When applied to diagnostic tests, specificity refers to the proportion of people who do not have a target disorder who have a negative test result.

Statistical significance (p-value) The likelihood of a result occurring by chance. By convention the level at which a result is said to be statistically significant is set at 5%, i.e. when there is less than a 5% probability that the result happened by chance, it is said to be statistically significant. This is usually written in the form of $p < 0.05$. The p-value does not, however, tell us how clinically important the result is.

Systematic review An overview of primary studies. The methods for the overview are made explicit and are reproducible, and steps are taken to eliminate or reduce bias.

Thick description A term used in qualitative research. A very detailed account of the methodological and interpretive strategy in the form of field notes.

Triangulation A strategy for strengthening the credibility of qualitative research. Multiple sources, methods, investigators or theories are used in combination to assess whether the findings are similar.

Truncation Used in searching electronic databases, truncation ensures that all terms that have the same text stem are found. For example a truncation mark at the end of 'child' will retrieve articles containing the terms child, childhood, childless, children, etc. The truncation mark may be an asterix (child*) or a dollar sign (child$) but varies according to the database provider.

Wildcard Similar to truncation, a wildcard is a character (in some databases it is a ?) that can be used to replace one or more characters. For example if the term 'p?ediatric' is searched, articles using the American spelling (pediatric) and articles using the British spelling (paediatric) will be retrieved.

Index